YOUNG, SICK, AND INVISIBLE

"The personal is political, and in *Young, Sick, and Invisible*,
Ania Bula drills down into both. Whether she's writing about medical
neglect, victim-blaming, invisibility, or woo and snake-oil medicine,
she tells her story with intensity, precision, and a clarity that resonates.
If you want better understanding and greater compassion
for people dealing with disabilities, I urge you to read it."

—Greta Christina, author of *The Way of the Heathen:
Practicing Atheism in Everyday Life*

"Living with illness and disability can be an isolating experience.
With her engaging, relatable writing Bula offers a kinship for those
who are searching. This is an important read."

—Kaleigh Trace, author of *Hot, Wet, and Shaking:
How I Learned to Talk About Sex*

"*Young, Sick, and Invisible* is an insightful look at one woman's journey
as she navigates the medical system, the expectations of others,
and her own place in the world. This book is hard to put down!"

—Angie Jackson, professional blogger

YOUNG, SICK, AND INVISIBLE

A Skeptic's Journey with Chronic Illness

Ania Bula

PITCHSTONE PUBLISHING
Durham, North Carolina

Pitchstone Publishing
Durham, North Carolina
www.pitchstonepublishing.com

10 9 8 7 6 5 4 3 2 1

Library of Congress Cataloging-in-Publication Data

Names: Bula, Ania, author.
Title: Young, sick, and invisible : a skeptic's journey with chronic illness
 / Ania Bula.
Description: Durham, North Carolina : Pitchstone Publishing, [2016]
Identifiers: LCCN 2015050304| ISBN 9781634310734 (paperback) | ISBN
 9781634310758 (pdf) | ISBN 9781634310765 (mobi)
Subjects: LCSH: Bula, Ania,—Health. | Crohn's
 disease—Patients—Ontario—Ottawa—Biography. | Psoriatic
 arthritis—Patients—Ontario—Ottawa—Biography. |
     Students—Ontario—Ottawa—Biography. | BISAC: BIOGRAPHY &
AUTOBIOGRAPHY /
 Women. | HEALTH & FITNESS / Women's Health.
Classification: LCC RC931.P76 B85 2016 | DDC 616.3/440092—dc23
LC record available at http://lccn.loc.gov/2015050304

To my amazing wife Alyssa Gonzalez,
without whose love and support this book would never have been written.

And

To the countless thousands of us living lives of invisible desperation.
You are not alone.

Contents

Poems

Introduction

Disability covers a wide range of conditions. It can be the result of an injury or illness, whether short-term or long-term. It can be something you're born with or something that develops over time. It can be constant, continuous, or relapsing and ever changing. It can be the cause or the result of other social issues. Everyone's experience with disability is different. Each type of disability may pose its own unique challenges, but almost all disabilities share certain commonalities, especially those that aren't obvious to the casual observer.

When your disability isn't written across your body for the world to see, there is a constant need to validate your need for self-care, or even your identity as someone who is disabled. Not being able to readily identify other people who are going through the same thing as you can be isolating. When you walk down the street, you can't know just from looking if someone else out there knows what it is like to feel your pain. You cannot know if someone will understand what you are going through. The isolation manifests as loneliness.

Healthy people don't know how to react to you. Some trivialize your experiences: either because they don't believe you are sick, or out of a desperate attempt to convince you that they are not judging you based on your disability. They point out that you don't look sick, or that other people they know with the same condition don't have nearly as much trouble with it as you do. Sometimes healthy people ignore you, pretend you don't exist, in an extreme enactment of the childhood injunction against staring.

Others jump to the opposite extreme and feel like they must keep reminding you of your weakness in order to keep you from harm. They overcompensate for their own discomfort by making it seem as though they are looking out for you. These are the people who are hyper alert for any sign that you are not at your best so that they can lecture you about taking it easy. Since you are never really at your best, this can start to make you feel useless. It can become grating as every single outing becomes peppered with the suggestion that maybe you shouldn't have gone out at all.

For most, it is difficult to strike that happy balance of treating a disabled individual like an independent human being—like any other adult—while also acknowledging that sometimes they might need to be more careful about what they eat or do, and understanding that perhaps they cannot go out as often as everyone else. As a result, you might feel as though you constantly have to justify yourself. That no, it is not just laziness that kept you in your pyjamas all day, or that you really do like their cooking but that yogurt keeps you up in pain all night. You worry that eventually everyone around you will be sick of trying and that you will be left friendless and alone.

Throughout all the self-doubt and loneliness, you are also struggling with managing your symptoms. No matter what your condition, exhaustion is a constant. Being sick takes a toll on your body and your mind, so that some days it can be an effort to get out of bed. Pain can be a constant companion, slowly draining your ability or willingness to even try.

Even as you are battling yourself and struggling to be a part of society, chronic illness acts as an invitation for everyone to comment on the likely causes of your disability, and possible treatments for it. Suddenly, everyone's aunt is an expert and everyone's fad diet a cure. You wade through a constant stream of ignorance and lies in a desperate attempt to stop the pain and find peace.

In my years of living with my various disorders I have been faith healed, poked, prodded, and stuffed with powders and magic potions, and now is my opportunity to tell everyone about it—so that my story might both help others, whether they are disabled or not, and help me, whether to cope with my past experiences or those to come.

Part 1: Psoriatic Arthritis

1 An Inauspicious Start

My story starts with a creak. Actually that's not entirely true, but the creak was the first instance that sticks out clearly in my mind. It was a Friday. I remember because on Fridays I had my chemistry course's laboratory section. It was my first year in university. Although not my first time being away from home, it was my first time completely on my own. It was in mid-September, long enough after my arrival for me to have gotten somewhat used to the whole situation, but still fresh enough to leave me uncertain.

On this particular Friday, my right hip began to make an odd creaking noise whenever I moved it. Although I noticed the sound and sensation, it wasn't unpleasant enough to elicit any major concern. My joints had always been strange and a source of discomfort. When a short while later the creaking turned into soreness, I still didn't think much of it. I was more excited about getting the chance to have lunch with my crush. I had no way of knowing that that creaking would be the start of a saga of pain, suffering, and disability that would change my life forever.

By the time my laboratory class had started, things had already progressed further. I could barely stand. My lower back felt as though someone had shoved a thick, rusty, hot needle through my spine. For the first time, I left most of the work to my lab partner as I tried to stay on one of the stools and not cry. I counted down the seconds for the class to end, until I could get out of there. As soon as our TA gave us permission to leave, I hobbled my way slowly to the university walk-in clinic in the building next door.

I don't remember exactly what I was thinking as I sat there. I wasn't expecting much. The clinic had a policy against prescribing opiates, which defined most pain meds. Unless something really caught the doctor's eye, I doubted there was anything they could do right away. Some part of me was counting down the seconds till I could get back to my dorm and take something for the pain, while another part of me was panicking over what could be causing this agony I was in.

The sudden onset, the extreme level of pain, and the difficulty with movement concerned the doctor on call. She apologized for her inability to prescribe me something for the pain and was relieved to hear that I already had some Naproxen back in my dorm. Earlier that same year, my family doctor back home in St. Catharines had prescribed Naproxen to treat the severe pain I experienced during my period. I did not take them regularly, only when the pain was bad enough to interfere with my everyday activities. The student health doctor suggested I go home, take the meds, and rest. In the meantime, she would arrange for a scan and some tests to figure out what the problem was.

I made my way home slowly, pulling myself along the walls and trying to keep myself from falling. The clinic was only a short five-minute walk from my residence. That day, the walk took me close to an hour. The sight of the three steps that led to the doors almost made me cry. I had finally made it. I took the painkillers immediately. The rest of the day, whenever I needed to walk somewhere , I used a chair as a walker. My father, who suffers from back problems, suggested that I sleep on my side with a pillow between my legs. The next morning, I woke up feeling better. Though I was still a bit stiff and sore, I filed away the episode as just an anomaly and mostly forgot about it.

Forgot that is, until the doctor called with my CT scan appointment a few months later. Although the pain was gone by then, something had to have caused the pain, and perhaps the scan would show something. This was not my first CT, having had one the year before after a bout with pancreatitis. The machine looks like a giant donut. You lie on a stretcher that moves back and forth until the technician completes the imaging. The whole procedure takes just a few minutes.

The clinic doctor called me back into the clinic a few weeks later. The scan had found some swelling in my sacroiliac joint, the one that connects your hip and pelvis to your spine. My right one was swollen enough to be noticeable even months after the pain had gone away. The doctor gave me a referral to a rheumatologist who would determine the cause of my swelling.

The rheumatologist was a really nice guy. We talked about the fact that he went to school with Sandra Oh. He did a quick medical history, asking whether arthritis was present in my family. He also asked about other conditions, such as psoriasis. His assumption was that the pain had been caused by even greater swelling in the joint earlier in the year. The Naproxen would have lowered the swelling and thus caused my miraculous recovery. I left the appointment with a diagnosis of psoriatic arthritis and a prescription for more nonsteroidal anti-inflammatories (NSAIDs) if I needed them. As it was explained to me, the arthritis was no big deal. It meant that I would have some pain from time to time and some stiffness in the mornings, but other than that it should have no effect on my everyday life.

Although at the time the diagnosis seemed mild, I was devastated. I was an eighteen-year-old girl with arthritis. I had never been on a date and had never even been kissed. I was convinced that if people knew that I was defective, I would be alone forever. In the typical melodrama of youth, I thought that this would be the worst thing to happen to me.

2 A Buggy Summer

Bed Bugs

Tiny little spots of darkness
An Army
Crawling across a desert
Of pale white
Raising mountains as they pass
Drinking from rivers of red
The ground moving
Like a giant sleeping
As the army marches across
The vast expanses
Sleep Tight
Don't Let the Bed Bugs Bite

That summer, I had been offered a job as a counselor at a children's camp. The training would start around mid-June, and the job itself would start in late June through the summer. I had left my residence hall and just moved into my first apartment: a room in the basement of an older couple's house. They had renovated their basement as an apartment for students, and it had multiple rooms, a large kitchen, laundry room, two toilets, and a shower.

I wanted the chance to experience freedom, so I decided to spend the weeks before camp in Ottawa. I found a temporary job at a Polish deli. There was a lot of standing around and lifting of heavy things, which left me feeling stiff at the end of my shift. On the second day, my boss brought up concerns that the other employees had had with my work; they had noticed me limping and were worried that it would affect my performance. I told my boss about my arthritis and she became even more concerned. She kept asking me if I was sure that I was up to the job. At the end of my third day, my family had a minor emergency that required me to return home to help take care of my little sister. Although I left for reasons other than my health, the feeling that my job had not been secure because I had a medical condition left a bad taste in my mouth.

Rather than seeing whether I could do the work with my condition, my boss's first reaction had been to doubt my abilities. I had done my work well, just with a limp, and the other employees had thought that justification enough to discuss my desirability as an employee with the boss. Even years later, whenever I go into the store, I have a hard time not feeling self-conscious and judged.

My time at home was pretty normal. The only occurrence of significance was being called in two weeks early to the camp, for a weekend's worth of training. The camp had arranged for all counselors to get lifeguard training to receive bronze medallion and the bronze cross certifications. In the coolness of May, the camp looked like a paradise. The cabins were like little hotels, with couches, running water, and the promise of air conditioners when the weather got warmer.

While there was some concern about how cold the water would be this early in the year, we were assured that it would be fine.

It wasn't. The water, when we jumped in, was freezing cold. But we're Canadians, we can take it, right? We proceeded with the course, making sure to stay moving to keep ourselves warm. It was an adventure. After training was over for the day, we swarmed the showers to warm ourselves up. Despite the heat of the cabin water, I could not completely dispel the cold that had seeped through my body. Moreover, I felt as though someone had placed a vise around my ribs. They felt similar to the time my sister bruised them when we were kids.

I went over the day in my mind and could not figure out when I might have injured them. When my back also started to twinge, I felt relief. Clearly the cold had set off my arthritis and all I needed to do was take my pain meds and relax for the evening. To that end, I excused myself from the campfire and stayed in the common room bundled up in a blanket reading. My ribs felt so tight that I could not fully catch my breath. I hoped that I would be better by the next morning, but I worried about what would happen when we went back into the water the next day.

Luckily, our instructors saw the light, and we were not forced back into the freezing water. Instead, they managed to find a local pool willing to open up their facilities for the training. We spent the day brushing up on the techniques necessary for pulling victims out of the water, performing artificial respiration, and so forth. By mid-day, my ribs still felt quite restricted, and I found it difficult to take full breaths. Although I had no trouble with the technical and lifesaving aspects of the training, I failed the speed and endurance test. Swimming thirty laps in fifteen minutes when you can't breathe is damn near impossible, though I came close, being only five laps short. I received one of the two certifications, and was not allowed to be the only counselor on duty during camp swims. More importantly, however, I felt the first impacts of my diagnosis of arthritis. I now knew I had limits, and while scary, they did not seem serious enough to be frightening.

We came back to the camp just a few weeks later for our job training. The weather had gotten much warmer, and we had to learn to cope with the realities of being in wetlands during the most humid months of the year. Another unexpected hardship was that the air conditioning systems had a pretty significant design flaw; rather than removing the humidity from the air while cooling, the ceiling vents accumulated thick droplets of water. These would rain down on us, the furniture, and the bedding. Our sleeping bags and bunks were almost permanently damp. We also discovered that, like many hotels throughout North America, this camp had been infested with bed bugs. I would wake up every morning with a new assortment of bites. It was only when they started showing up in places where no mosquito would have access did I realize what was going on. When the bites started swelling to the size of quarters, I realized that I was allergic to them.

Being a camp counselor is an incredibly intense job. We had to wake up early in the morning to get ourselves ready before we woke the kids up to get them going as well. You are responsible for the health, happiness, and overall well-being of a whole group of kids, who all seem determined to get themselves into trouble. For all the energy they have, you need to have that much more just to keep everything and everyone in control.

You cannot go to sleep until all of your kids, who are at a peak state of excitement, do. We would often stay up until 1 or 2 a.m., and then be back up at 6 in the morning to start it all over again. Eating becomes an issue as you face the exact same meals with each successive camp rotation. Ninety percent of the lunches and dinners were chicken. By the time I left the camp, just the smell of chicken was enough to make me sick.

For the first few weeks of camp, we had not managed to work out how to take our breaks. Given the sleep deprivation, malnutrition, physical intensity, stress, damp beds, and bed bugs, it is not surprising that after a month and a half my body gave out. I started feeling very sick. Instead of a fever, though, my body temperature was over a full degree lower than normal. My hip and lower back had started bothering me and no amount of NSAIDs could make it fully go away.

I started avoiding the more physically intensive activities. I couldn't force myself to walk down to the zip line and mountain climbing areas. I traded with other counselors to take over their farm and art sections. And still my situation proceeded to get worse. Finally, just a few days before my birthday, I had to give up. I quit my job and went back home. I hoped that after a few weeks of rest and relaxation I would recover enough for my lower body pain not to bother me anymore.

When I quit my job, the supervisors were upset that I had not brought up my concerns regarding my hip and back pain sooner. They would have been willing to work around my disability, they said. By this point, however, it was clear to me that even if I were excused from all the physically intense activities, the stress and inability to sleep and eat would continue wreaking havoc with my body. What's more, the deli that summer had taught me an important lesson: being open about your disability puts you at risk for losing your job. Better to quit on my own terms than be fired for something I cannot control.

3 Looking for Answers

The few weeks of rest in St. Catharines, before the start of the new semester, helped me regain some of my health, though my leg still ached pretty consistently. Although the scans suggested that any problems were being caused by my hip specifically, the pain often extended throughout my entire leg. Sometimes the focus was the hip, such as when sitting or shifting position. But at other times, it felt as though my femur was about to shatter, and my whole leg seemed to be on fire with agony. Luckily, I had an appointment scheduled with my rheumatologist in late September. I returned to Ottawa at the beginning of September, ready for class and looking forward to getting the help I needed to make the pain go away.

As the days passed, the pain got worse. Imagine that every time you sit down you feel as though your hip is popping out of its joint. That it takes ten minutes for the pain to stop once your joint becomes accustomed to its new position. Then when you stand, it feels as though you are forcing it back into place. This is what it felt like every day, with nearly every movement. I began to wonder if perhaps I had actually injured myself at the camp. With my appointment at the rheumatologist still some days away, and concerned that I would need X-rays, I decided to go to the walk-in clinic.

The moment the doctor I saw heard I had arthritis, she sent me on my way, telling me to take my painkillers and to call my rheumatologist. I was annoyed that she hadn't even bothered to examine my hip, or question why I had chosen to come see her rather than my specialist. Having arthritis doesn't magically prevent me from being injured. In fact, one could argue that impairment to my joints could make me more accident prone.

Disappointed and frustrated over having wasted my time at the clinic, I waited for my upcoming appointment with the specialist. When the time finally came, I told my rheumatologist about the pain I was experiencing. He seemed unconcerned. With the high-intensity summer that I had had, he suggested that I might have somehow sprained my hip. He prescribed me a cane and sent me on my way. I was relieved to find an answer, and I picked up my stylish new cane—black, with foam handle and adjustable height (woo baby!)— at the pharmacy downstairs. I figured that after a few weeks of taking the weight off my leg, I would be back to normal; no big deal. My father, when I called him to get help with purchasing the cane, made a joke about being careful, since "Cain dis-Abeled the world after all."

4 Learned Helplessness

Over the course of the next few weeks, rather than getting better, things got progressively worse. Soon my whole right leg was on fire with never-ending pain. Every step made me feel as though my tibia would shatter beneath me. I swear that I could feel the pressure fractures forming. In the mornings, my body was so stiff that even the lightest pressure caused pain. At night, falling asleep was almost impossible, as I struggled to find the least painful position. When my leg started losing feeling and giving out beneath me, I realized I couldn't keep dismissing my symptoms as just a normal hip sprain. I realized that they indicated something more severe and that I needed to have it checked out.

With the loss of feeling and support in the limb, not to mention the jumps in pain, I wondered about the possibility of a pinched nerve, a blood clot, or something else. It was even suggested that I might have bone tuberculosis. This was somewhat plausible as a relative had been suffering from TB when I last visited family in Poland, and other people in our community were possible "healthy" carriers. I finally decided to go see a doctor to discuss my worries.

This being my second year in university, I did not have a doctor in Ottawa. When I was in school, the majority of people did not have one. There was a deficit of general practitioners who were accepting new patients, and I was unfamiliar with Ottawa outside of the university and the immediate vicinity of my apartment. Thankfully, the university provided a health clinic to meet basic student needs. Although I had had negative experiences before at this clinic—some very negative—I had also had positive experiences, like with the doctor who helped me get diagnosed with arthritis.

I was no stranger to pain. Before my diagnosis, I had had mysterious joint pain for as long as I could remember, particularly in high school. I can clearly remember several occasions where I spent anywhere from a few days to up to a week limping. On multiple occasions I brought it up with my parents, only to be told that all I had to do was lose weight. On the few occasions when I managed to get an appointment with a doctor, it often involved one of my parents asking the doctor to tell me about how all my issues would be solved if I lost weight.

Eventually, I didn't even need my parents' presence to get such a response. It seemed to be firmly ingrained in doctors' minds that any complaint that could be explained away as being the result of fat, should be. The closest I came to being taken seriously was when my doctor diagnosed me with patellofemoral pain syndrome. I often wonder how much pain I could have saved myself, how much of my eventual disability I could have spared myself from, had I pushed past the preconceptions set up by my parents. It is easy to get caught in the trap of what could have been, of blame, and of self-hate. So why didn't I push past it? Why didn't I self-advocate and demand that I be taken seriously? Because to some extent not being taken seriously by doctors, being told that I was overreacting, was conditioned early.

When my family moved from Saskatoon to St. Catharines, we had a doctor who was convinced I was a hypochondriac. Before we moved, I had been experiencing a consistent cough. My parents did what any parent would reasonably do: they gave me Triaminic. The coughing was so bad, however, that I kept bringing up the syrup. Eventually I was diagnosed with allergies. After more time, it was finally discovered that I had asthma. Those coughing fits signaled the start of asthma attacks. Despite the diagnosis being confirmed by an allergist, and there being a known link between asthma and upper-respiratory infections, my family doctor still thought that I was faking.

I was a klutzy kid who was often bullied. I would trip and fall so often, my family would joke that I should walk around with elbow and knee pads. I often joked that I must have been made of rubber. With how often I fell, it is pretty shocking that I only ever managed to break a bone once—I fell on some ice, and fractured my left wrist right underneath the growth plate. When I went to the ER, the doctor couldn't see the hairline fracture on X-ray because of its location. Due to all my symptoms, however, he was certain that the bone was fractured and put my wrist in a splint. So convinced that I was a hypochondriac, my family doctor took off the splint when I went in for a follow-up two weeks later. To this day, I get twinges of pain in the same spot where the fracture had been.

It became a connection in my mind: complain about a concern too frequently and you won't be believed. The only way to have a concern taken seriously is to make sure that it had not been mentioned in some time.

By the time my family switched doctors, the idea that I was a faker had been firmly ingrained in my parents' mind. One particular event stands out: my father and I had gone out to restaurant, and we ended up overeating, and my stomach had that unpleasantly stretched feeling. The next morning the stretched feeling had not gone away. Throughout the day, I had a hard time standing up straight, and I felt as though my energy was draining out. When the pain got so bad that I had to take a break from cleaning the kitchen, my mother accused me of being lazy. I was often berated for doing anything other than cleaning. When the next day I still felt that continuing pain in my stomach, I knew I had to see a doctor. I walked a few blocks to the clinic near my house. The close proximity meant that I did not have to rely on my parents to get myself there.

When the doctor saw me, I was given a referral to the ER. My dad drove me and we got fast tracked. Soon I was seeing a doctor who assured me that everything would be fine and that I could probably go home as soon as the blood test results came in. Half an hour later, he came into the room saying there had been a change of plans and I was being admitted. I had pancreatitis—inflammation of the pancreas indicated by an increase in my lipase levels. I spent the next seven days knocked out on Demerol, on a starvation diet. I missed a much-anticipated trip to Stratford to see a well-known Shakespearean actor in his final role in *Macbeth*. My mother felt terrible about not believing me. Unfortunately her remorse and lesson from that experience never seemed to impact future behavior.

5 Losing Faith

When I finally made the decision to go to the walk-in clinic to see whether the extreme pain I was experiencing might have a cause other than my arthritis, I was particularly worried about a blood clot. Between my weight and my relative inactivity due to the pain in my leg, I was concerned that I might have developed a clot that was contributing to the pain. The doctor I saw was a very pleasant young woman. She listened to me, concerned, and then stepped out for a moment. When she came back into the room, she said words that shocked me so badly that I still remember them to this day: "I think it is something serious, but I don't know what tests to run so I'm just going to send you home."

Imagine being in that situation. You are worried about your health. You think something serious might be going on. Possibilities of blood clots, tumors, nerve problems, etc. are dancing through your head. You go to a doctor to find out what might be wrong, to either put your mind at ease or at least give you an answer about why you feel the way you do. Instead the doctor legitimizes your panic, but refuses to do anything about it. They send you home. Send you to go back, answerless, to that pain and that concern. No suggestion of going to the hospital. No request for time. Just washing their hands of you because they don't know what tests to run and cannot be bothered to try and figure it out.

I was devastated, in a panic, and angry. At that moment, these feelings were just beginning to make themselves known. By the end of the ordeal, they would become familiar old friends.

I decided to skip my classes the next day and head to the ER. The doctor had said that she thought it was something serious, and at this point there was no good reason to wait. At that time, the ER in Ottawa had a policy of asking patients how they got there, the idea being that if you didn't get there under your own power then it must be more serious than people who got there via the bus or driving. I had taken a taxi, which apparently counted as getting there under my own power. The waiting room was poorly organized. The chairs were hard, uncomfortable, and poorly designed for people who might be in pain and would be waiting a very long time. The whole arrangement was reminiscent of school plays held in elementary school gyms. This was before the ER reorganized, and so all the waiting was done in this one large room.

After a four-hour wait without being called in to see a doctor, I was sent for X-rays. Two hours after that, I was still waiting to see a doctor. After eight hours, I had still not seen a doctor and was getting desperate. The chairs had left me with even more pain than I had had before. When I had arrived at the hospital it was daytime; by this point it was already evening. I began to wonder if I was going to be spending the whole night there in the waiting room. Eventually a nurse took pity on me and called me over to her desk: "I shouldn't be showing you this. I am not a doctor and so I am not allowed to offer diagnoses, but I thought you might want to see your X-rays."

I understood the implied disclaimer and we sat down and looked at the X-rays. She pointed out that my right hip had half the cartilage of the other hip. This in itself pointed out that I had some serious inflammation at the joint. What was more alarming was what she pointed out along the head of the femur. Normally, the head is smooth and round. In my case, however, the bone was jagged. It was clear that whatever was going on was doing serious, permanent damage to my leg. This, finally, was the answer to my pain. Now I just needed to know what was causing it.

I went back to the waiting room to wait for the doctor. After another hour I was finally called in. The doctor came into the room, barely looking at me: "Okay, so I took a look at your X-rays and there is no evidence of cancer. Looks like there is nothing to worry about."

If you've ever had a computer, you have probably seen the infamous blue screen of death. When I heard those words, I felt as though my head was flashing that screen. I crashed. I had been waiting all day by this point. I was tired, in pain, and had just wasted hours, only to have this doctor claim that the draining, excruciating pain I had been experiencing was *nothing to worry about.* This, after seeing for myself that something serious was going on—cartilage doesn't disappear by itself, and a bone certainly doesn't become jagged without reason.

"I wasn't worried about cancer . . ."

"Oh?"

"No. I wanted to know what was causing this extreme pain I'm in. I can barely walk and it feels like my leg is shattering when I do. I'm losing feeling in the leg as well."

"Well, there was nothing on your X-rays that were of any concern."

I was astounded. I couldn't believe what he was claiming. I wanted him to explain what I had seen on my X-rays, so I asked him to show them to me. The doctor blustered for a bit, mumbling something about giving me a Percocet, but by this point I had had enough. I wasn't leaving until I saw those X-rays. He took me to a back room with a light board and put my X-rays up to it. Blown up, the difference between the two joints, my left and right hips, was even more painfully obvious. Frustrated, I pointed this out.

"What about the fact that my right hip joint has less than half the cartilage of my left joint."

The doctor leaned in close, "Oh, hey! You're right!"

I felt deflated and exhausted. I knew that the best I was going to get out of this was a couple of extra-strength painkillers and a headache. Defeated, I took the pills he gave me and headed home.

6 Living with Chronic Pain

When you are young and in pain, there is a tendency by most others to think that you are overreacting. They can't believe that someone who has not even seen their twentieth year could be in pain that severe. Chronic pain in particular is not something that happens to young people. They believe that is has to be a cry for attention or, more nefariously, an attempt to get drugs. This is the experience I found through countless encounters with doctors during the first months of my hip problem. After the ER, I went back to my rheumatologist. He gave me some muscle relaxants and new anti-inflammatories to try and sent me on my way. I don't know if he ever saw the X-rays done by the hospital, though he never thought to order his own.

Unfortunately, the muscle relaxants had a side effect: in the mornings after taking them, I would wake up with my muscles feeling so stiff that I could barely move. I soon gave up taking them.

The new NSAIDs had an unfortunate tendency to dissolve into powder if you didn't swallow them fast enough. On multiple occasions, the powder would catch on the back of my throat and make me vomit. Most mornings, it was a choice of whether I wanted to feel sick for a few hours or be in pain. Often being sick won out and I would take them, trying hard to swallow as fast as possible. From time to time, I would have to spit out the powder rather than try to swallow it. I soon learned that I had a much easier time swallowing if I used pop to wash them down. With water, I could taste the bitterness much more.

At least the pills had some effect. On the days when I was able to keep them down, I would have a brief hour-long window where I would feel a little better. Often that hour of time would coincide with the moment when I was walking through the busiest corridor at the university. From time to time, I would test a theory. I would pick up my cane and do a small, low-intensity dance to see if anyone would notice. Only one person ever did. A young man, who turned around violently to see if he had seen right and promptly fell over from turning too fast.

People can get used to pain. It might seem odd and counterintuitive, but it's true. When you go through periods of intense pain that lasts weeks, or even months, it becomes a part of the background noise. It is like the difference between a conversation you have in your home versus one you have in a crowded restaurant. You still manage to have the conversation, but in the restaurant you have to work a little harder to hear all of it. From time to time, the noise swells and you miss some of what is being said. At other times, there is a lull and the conversation comes through crystal clear. Similarly, you have to struggle a bit more to experience all you can of life, but you are still plugging away. From time to time, the pain will swell in such a way as to make you have to stop. You can't help it—the background noise just gets too loud. At other times, something great happens and you have a short lull in the pain. During this lull you can experience more.

Sometimes, you go a little overboard by trying to rush into life all at once and, in doing so, bring on the sharp rises in pain faster. But no matter what, the pain, the background noise, is always there. While it might not bother you while you are distracted from it, there are moments when the background noise interferes with your activities. Sleeping becomes more difficult. You toss and turn all night, trying to find that exact position that will quiet everything down.

Most nights, I would sleep in a strange half-sideways, half-on-my-back position, held together by cleverly placed pillows. Moving at night was out of the question. Doing so would result in being woken by a sharp stab of pain. Sometimes, in order to forget about the pain, I would inflict some other, different pain to distract me from the larger one. I would scratch something, or dig my nails into my palms, anything to take the edge off. There were many nights when sleep would evade me.

Eventually, the lack of sleep would catch up with me and I would have to skip a class or two to try to bring my energy back up. I would spend many hours in bed. When I did manage to fall asleep, my dreams were plagued by pain. I would wake up as exhausted as I had felt the night before. When those moments got particularly bad, I would try the ER again. I did so in the hopes that this time, finally, I would meet the doctor who would figure out why I was in so much agony.

On the nights and days when I lay in bed overwhelmed by pain, I would focus on it. I would let it consume me utterly until I could feel every tendril of it. I would imagine it as yellow. Once I held it completely in my mind, I would imagine compressing it like a child does with a piece of cotton candy. I would compress it and compress it until it reached the size of a pea. All that pain concentrated in one spot. Then, with all of my concentration I would push it slowly down my leg, into my foot, then into my toe, and then finally I would work on pushing it out of me. The fierce concentration I was using in this process allowed me to fool myself, if only for half a second, that the pain was gone. I would hope that if I managed to fool myself often enough, I would be able to fall asleep.

More effective was masturbation. I would bring myself to the edge then ride it, letting the cascading waves of pleasure drown out the pain. When even that didn't work, I would play with the pain, embrace it until it became intertwined with my desire. I made my pain my pleasure. I may be one of the only people in the world who actively tried to induce masochistic tendencies in myself. It worked to an extent, but—and this was the case with just the straight masturbation or meditation—only if I didn't move at all. A single shift of my body would send lances of pain to my hip and ruin everything. Context is everything, and no amount of self-determination, willpower, stubbornness, or anything could make the pain experienced during movement anything other than unbearable.

7 Not So Invisible

Walking with the cane identified me as someone with a disability. While it was just a bit of metal and plastic, in practice it was a wall between me and normalcy. When you have a cane, or a wheelchair, or any other aid, you are automatically identified as other, as different. No matter what you do, you will never fully be part of the group.

In some ways, living with a disability is like living constantly in a box or a bubble. You can see the outside world, and interact with people, but there exists a permanent barrier between you and everyone else— one you cannot get through no matter how hard you try. This barrier is not actually imposed by the disability itself, but by social attitudes surrounding disability.

This became obvious when a certain group of friends became obsessed with trying to do everything for me. One in particular would interrupt what I was saying so that she could run ahead to open the door for me. While at first her help and concern felt nice, eventually it became grating. It got to the point where I became irrationally angry every time she opened the door for me. You see, she thought she was doing a good deed and she expected to be praised for it —*Oh, look at the nice person, holding the door open for the poor little crippled girl.* In actuality, what she and others were doing was reinforcing this idea that I was completely helpless—that without their help, concern, and intervention, I would be trapped.

What made it worse for me was the fact that, to some extent, they were right. We live in a society where accessibility is not the standard; it's the exception. We live in a society where, if you help me against my will, I have to smile and thank you because you were just trying to be nice. Where I don't have a right to my pride or my independence, because I am different and everyone else is being accommodating to my difference. The world is doing me a favor by allowing me to have some of the same experiences as anyone else, and to expect real equality is just being selfish. When they call me a disabled person, what they mean is that my personhood has been disabled, because I no longer have a right to my own body, to make decisions for myself, or to be treated as an independent human adult. Oftentimes, the biggest barriers faced by disabled people are not those imposed by our bodies or minds. They are the ones imposed by others.

Think about how people react to successful persons with disabilities: she won an Olympic medal, a feat that is really impressive for a *blind* person. She made millions through a brilliant invention, but what is really impressive is that she is in a *wheelchair*. They look so much like successful people despite being *damaged*. The way people talk about differently abled people smacks very much of being given a cookie. Oh, look at that! You got into university just like everyone else, but because you are also crippled in some way, here have a cookie because you are *special*. It comes from a good place, but reeks of condescension. Ultimately, the message is that no one expects anything of us, so when we end up being like anyone else, that is *impressive*. Everything you do, no matter how impressive or even how underwhelming, is seen through the lens of disability. Praise is tinged with pity, with the belief that even though you do something outstanding, deep down you must really only desire to be like everyone else. She made millions, but she would trade it all just to be able to walk, or see, or hear, or anything else.

8 What Is Normal?

The concept of normalcy is confusing, and ultimately harmful. Normalcy implies that there is a standard, a norm, for all experience and behavior. The normal human being can see, hear, walk, move in a certain way, speak a certain way, act a certain way. Where this concept runs into problems is that it doesn't hold up under examination. No two human beings see in exactly the same way. We have long known, for example, that the perception of color changes from person to person. The green I see is not exactly the same as the green you see and so on. We also have varying degrees of sightedness. If this were not the case, we would not have so many people who wear glasses. Our concept of normalcy is that you can see this clearly at a certain distance. For the sake of convenience sake, it is called 20/20. A close examination of our society, however, would probably reveal that the majority of the population does not correspond to this criteria, that in terms of population, the percentage who can actually see 20/20 is actually quite small. Despite this, however, our concept of normalcy is still centered on 20/20 vision.

We've already seen the way the concept of normalcy backfires in other aspects of our society. It was once thought in Western society, for example, that the normal human being was white-skinned. As much as we would like to think otherwise, this concept of normalcy is still prevalent in our society. This concept is what continues to influence racism: I don't have to treat people who are not white as human beings because they are not *normal*.

Other examples of normalcy include sexual orientation, sexual expression and desire, gender expression, and more. Time and time again, concepts of what is normal backfire and are ultimately shown to be untrue. People who are completely straight and interested in "normal" sex, and fit completely into the established normal expressions of gender and gender roles, are ultimately rare, if they truly exist at all. Think about that. A personified model of normalcy doesn't actually exist. There is no completely normal person out there. Moreover, what is considered normal changes from one society to the next. If normalcy existed as a standard, it would be the same regardless of whether you are presently in society A or society B.

As long as we maintain these standards of what is normal, we will continue to run into systems of oppression simply because the real human norm is *diversity*.

This is not to say that we shouldn't celebrate the accomplishments of people with disabilities or other minorities. Their accomplishments deserve to be lauded the same way as anyone else's. Rather, my problem with many of these stories lies in that they ignore an important truth—the reason their stories are impressive is because **our society is not accessible**. The stories are not about celebrating accomplishments but rather about easing our own guilt. They are accessibility's version of the Republican's bootstraps story. By showing how one person can overcome the obstacles we as a society have thrown at them, we can pretend that those obstacles really aren't all that bad or even that they don't exist. That anyone complaining about those obstacles is just lazy, or looking for an excuse, or a "professional victim."

In many cases, the stories of people with disabilities really are impressive, but they shouldn't have to be. In a society where we have incredible capabilities for technology and innovation, the ability of a person to succeed should not be limited because of a physical impairment. It is not our physical conditions that disable us, but rather society itself.

If you ask most able-bodied persons whether our societies are accessible, most will answer yes. After all, elevators exist almost everywhere and we see ramps all the time, so clearly accessibility must not be an issue. If you think this way, I offer you a challenge. For the next week, every time that you had to use even so much as one stair in order to get somewhere, I would like you to put a dollar in a jar. This includes going to a store, coffee shop, classroom, workplace, restaurant, event, house, apartment, anywhere really. For one week, every time you have to use an inaccessible entrance in order to not be late, or simply for convenience, because the accessible entrance is far out of the way, I want you to put a dollar into the jar. Every time you encounter an entrance that doesn't have automatic capabilities or that has a broken handicapped button, I want you to put a dollar in the jar. I guarantee that if you are aware and honest, by the end of the week, you will have an impressive sum of money.

When we discuss accessibility there is a tendency to think of only certain types of disabilities. As long as we cater only to those, we consider society as a whole to be accessible. Ultimately, however, that leads people who don't fall within those specific categories to be disadvantaged. I will give you an example from personal experience: during the period where I had to walk with a cane, I had a hard time using the stairs. Going up stairs was painful as it engaged my hip more than many other activities. Given the choice, I preferred to take an elevator. More often than not, however, the elevators were placed in areas far out of the way. This would force me to have to walk for longer periods of time, a process that was also extremely painful.

Ottawa residents might be familiar with the UOttawa Campus bus station. It is one of two transit way stations that service the University of Ottawa campus. The campus stop services the science and engineering buildings. The eastbound stop is across from the university buildings. Rather than risking students having to cross a street filled with buses, they built an underpass. There is an elevator on the eastbound side allowing access to the upstairs station; however, in order to get down to the underpass, there are no elevators. Instead, the university has built a curving ramp on either side of the long stairs leading down. There are also steeper stairs that lead directly from the westbound station to the underpass.

For someone with a wheelchair, access is assured with the ramp. For someone like me, however, the choice is either going several meters out of my way, followed by a long trek down a ramp, or braving steep stairs. Moreover, the steeper stairs next to the westbound station also happen to be closed off most of the time in winter. This may not seem like a big deal, but the choice to add a long ramp rather than an elevator means more pain for me and anyone else in a similar situation. It means when taking the shorter route up the stairs, you are also taking a risk that your leg will give out on a step. I've had that happen. I know what it is like to have your leg suddenly stop working right when you've reached the most dangerous height. I am so familiar with it in fact that, even today, when my leg giving out is no longer as big a concern, I still experience a moment of severe vertigo and flashback when standing at the top of a flight of stairs.

9 It Continues

My visits to the hospital had been fruitless, and I continued to drag myself along with a cane. Although falling over or collapsing was a serious concern—especially when it happened in the middle of crossing the street—there were moments when it provided amusement as well.

One particular morning sticks out in my mind: my sister went to a French school, like I did. Our parents are big fans of language education and the boost that it gives to future career and living options. They themselves, however, do not speak French. From time to time, they called me for help with my sister's homework or pronunciation. My parents also know I am not a big fan of early mornings. As a result I have an assumption that if I receive a phone call between the hours of 11 p.m. at night and 9 a.m., that something terrible must have happened. So you can imagine my concern when I get woken up at six in the morning with my cellphone ringing across the room. I jumped out of bed in a panic, forgetting that walking without a cane wasn't among my abilities. I collapsed to the ground, and then when I tried to stand up, I tripped and fell again. Giving up, I dragged myself across the floor by my hands and grabbed the phone. Out of breath, in pain, and in fear, I answered the phone only to hear my father's voice: "What's the French word for 'cow'?"

Sometime around the start of the Christmas season, an old family friend was throwing a party, and my parents had decided to drive up to Ottawa to attend it. At the party were several friends from Saskatoon whom we hadn't seen in some years. Among them was an old doctor friend who was like a grandfather to me. Over the course of the evening, the doctor friend managed to corner me to ask what was going on with my leg. He wanted to know why someone as young and as comparatively healthy as me was having such a hard time walking and moving. We talked, and he took me seriously. He suggested I go back to my rheumatologist and request a medication called Enbrel. It was guaranteed, he said, to help me with my pain.

In the meantime, over Christmas, I went back to the Niagara region to spend the holidays with family. At the time, my parents were pretty irritated with the fact that I was using a cane. To their mind, this was nothing more than another attempt at getting attention. Clearly I was looking for any excuse to be lazy.

One of my mother's favorite techniques for getting her own way is to prey on the vulnerabilities of her opponents. At nineteen years of age, I had never been kissed, on a real date, or even knowingly been courted in any way. The addition of the cane meant that I was even more self-conscious than usual about my lack of a love life. It was a weakness my mother tried to exploit to her advantage in trying to convince her daughter to stop faking it: "No man will ever love you if you are crippled."

This wasn't the first time I had heard some variation of the "no man" threat. Previously it had focused on my weight, with the understanding that no man would love me as long as I continued to be fat. This new twist was ultimately nothing new. Usually, I would mostly ignore the comment in that moment, only to have it haunt me for months afterward. This time however, I was already dealing with the fear that if I was sick, in addition to not being conventionally attractive, the possibility of me dying alone was all the more likely. Already in my head, the fear of being a sixty-year-old virgin who had never been kissed persisted. I had some variation of this fear ever since I received my initial diagnosis. To hear this from my mother, the person who is supposed to be a source of love, understanding, and support, broke something in me.

I returned to Ottawa and to a meeting with my rheumatologist. I brought up the recommendation I had received from my family friend, about Enbrel. My doctor was familiar with the medication, but insisted that at my age, such a strong course of treatment was unwise. I didn't know it at the time, but the drug is an immunosuppressant. It works by limiting the antibody that is responsible for attacking the joints in psoriatic arthritis ("PA") patients. My doctor mentioned how people make antibodies against certain treatments. He was sure that if he prescribed it now, by the time I was sixty years old, when I might need it even more, it wouldn't work for me.

Thinking back now, I wish I had pressed the point. By the time I'm sixty years old, they will surely have new medications. Moreover, considering the state of inflammation in my leg, worrying about something taking place forty years from now was tantamount to worrying that the carpet might go out of style in a house that is currently on fire.

Instead my doctor recommended steroid shots, particularly cortisol, to be injected into my hip and back. I was on board, and reminded my doctor that I had an allergy to fluoroscopic dye. Since the procedure he was recommending would involve some sort of imaging, I wanted to make sure that he didn't book me for anything that would require exposure to that particular type of dye. When the hospital called a few days later to book the appointment, I repeated my concerns. I was assured that it wouldn't be a problem.

I had discovered my allergy when I had been admitted to the hospital with pancreatitis some years earlier. As part of my CT scan, they injected me with dye in order to see what they needed to see. Fluoroscopic dye creates a feeling of warmth when injected, and many people feel like they are about to pee when they get it. After they injected me with the dye, I was convinced that I had peed myself. The warmth was very intense and I couldn't believe that I hadn't in fact had an accident. As soon as the scan was over I ran to the washroom. It was there that I discovered that, although I had not urinated, something else was going on. My eye was swollen. It was so swollen that it looked as though I had been hit with a baseball bat. The nurses rushed to get me some Benadryl, and the swelling went down. While the whole experience wasn't overly traumatic, I was warned that facial swelling could potentially mean something more serious. I was cautioned to avoid the dye in the future, and also to avoid shellfish, which contains the same protein.

When I arrived at my appointment, I was a little nervous. It was potentially the chance for me to feel better. If this worked, I might be able to walk again, and I might be able to stop missing classes because of my lack of sleep. The possibility of an end to pain was overwhelming. I was brought into a separate room in radiology and the nurse explained the procedure to me: they would use an X-ray to find my joints and inject me with a steroid. The steroid in question would stop the swelling and the pain would go away. I would be getting two shots, one in my hip and another in my lower back, in the sacroiliac joint.

I agreed to all of it, and then the doctor arrived and the x-ray was set up. Just as we were about to begin, the nurse said she needed to give me a quick injection.

"You're going to feel a little warm, but don't worry, that's normal."

I snapped to attention. "That's not fluoroscopic dye is it?" I asked in a panic.

"Yes . . ." She answered, confused.

I explained that I had let the hospital and my doctor know on multiple occasions that I was allergic to it. Again and again, I had asked them to make sure that I wasn't booked for a procedure where its use was necessary. The doctor looked at me, frustrated, and explained that the only other way to make sure the injection went in the right place, without using the dye, was to get a CT, which could give a cross-section without the dye and give an accurate depiction of where the needle was.

There was something about the way that the doctor was talking to me that made me feel as though he believed I was making it up. I wasn't, though, and so the doctor was forced to come up with a solution. He agreed to give me the hip injection guided just by X-ray right away. For the injection in my spine, however, I would have to wait a few weeks until they could book the CT. I agreed. Some relief now was better than having to wait months. It would also give me some idea if the steroids were going to work. All in all, I was just glad to finally have doctors taking my pain seriously.

They inserted a needle into my hip joint and started pumping me full of steroids. It didn't hurt, but felt more like knocking, *thud, thud, thud,* as they injected the stuff into me. Over the next couple days my pain lessened dramatically. All that remained was some stiffness in my lower back and leg. I rejoiced. I assumed that the remaining stiffness would go away once I got the second injection. In the meantime, I tried to get back to normal life.

10 Getting Back to Normal?

I got a job at a pharmacy. I played *Dance Dance Revolution*. I went out dancing. I started to participate in normal activities that were far beyond me when I had been in pain. I didn't notice that things were still wrong. Or, rather, I made a strong effort to ignore them. A four-hour shift at the pharmacy left my back feeling too stiff. My legs and feet would get tired too fast. I remember that in my interview with the pharmacy, I was asked point blank if I thought my arthritis would impede my ability to do my work. I was sure it wouldn't.

After months of pain, I could walk again, surely nothing could go wrong for me anymore. It was my manager who pointed out just how strange the way I bent over was. When I needed to bend down, I had to stick my leg straight out behind me. It was something I simply hadn't noticed.

When the hospital called next, it wasn't for my second injection, but rather a referral for an endoscopy—a procedure that involved inserting a camera down my throat. They wanted to make sure that there weren't any other underlying issues. Apparently with arthritis, especially psoriatic arthritis, it is very common for people to have a secondary autoimmune disorder, so checking out my digestive system was standard operating procedure. The endoscopy showed nothing of concern. There was a vague reference to the idea that I should get a colonoscopy at some point, but it was all low priority.

During this time, people started giving me recommendations, speculating about my condition and what might have caused it or could make it go away. Their suggestions were still mild enough that I wasn't overly bothered. Many had to do with food: I was told that tomatoes, tea, coffee, and various other foods cause inflammation.

Despite the stiffness, I was optimistic and looked forward to the next injection. If one had made such an improvement, surely two would mean the end to all my problems. I would be better! I would be normal again!

More than a month after my initial injection I got the appointment for the next one. Since we couldn't use the contrast dye, we would need to use a CT scan in order to make sure the needle went into the right place. I was told to lie flat on my stomach while they marked out where it should go. They inserted the needle, put me back through the machine to check placement, made adjustments, until finally everything was in the right place. After that, the injection was made and I was sent home.

The day after my procedure I wasn't feeling well and stayed home. I was a little sore, but figured that it was to be expected after having had a needle in my spine.

Two days later, I couldn't walk. I got up to go to the bathroom and fell on my face. I lay there for a few minutes, my whole body wracked with pain. Unless you've been there it is nearly impossible to explain the feeling of absolute helplessness, of vulnerability, of desperation when you are lying on the floor because you have lost the ability to walk and you have to pee.

I dragged myself. I don't know how, but I dragged myself to the hospital. I grabbed a wheelchair and rolled myself up to the window and told them that two days before I had had an injection into my spine and now I couldn't walk.

They sent me to urgent care. I had some expectation that out of fear of liability I would perhaps get a chance to see the doctor faster. I thought that, perhaps out of fear of what might have happened to my spine, they might take it seriously. Instead, I waited. I waited for close to six hours before a doctor saw me and took a look at my back and at the injection site. The doctor must have been with me for less than five minutes. He told me that sometimes a little swelling occurs after such an injection and that I would feel better in a day or two. He sent me home.

I was not better in a day or two. In fact, in that time things got worse. The pain would not subside and I couldn't get out of bed except to go to the bathroom. I ordered food because I couldn't stand to cook for myself. Two days after I had gone to the hospital, I tried again. Only this time, I went to a different one. This time, after I dragged myself up the stairs from my basement apartment, to the waiting cab, I went to a hospital at the other end of town. The driver was nice enough to get me a wheelchair so that

I could wheel myself in. When I got to the reception, I broke down and cried.

In all this time, I had always tried to put on a brave face, whether in the ER, among friends, to teachers . . . If I cried, I did so privately. I was in pain, but I wouldn't let myself cry. By this point, I had reached my breaking point. I couldn't do it anymore. I cried. I saw the doctor relatively quickly after that. They gave me an injection of morphine and antinausea medication. When the doctor heard that I had had an injection in my spine less than a week prior he was very concerned. He sent me home with a bottle of morphine and the promise that he would get me an MRI within a week.

11 Breaking Point

Ode to Psoriatic Arthritis
(An author's pain)

I stand proud
But bent
Cut down in my prime
Searing pain shooting through me
My legs giving out
No one understands my pain
Ridicule me
Pity me
But never understand me
They see not my pain
They see only my age
My inexperience
Believe that I lie

I take a step and fall
My whole life flashing before me
A vast expanse of pain
A lonely space

I disguise myself with smiles
Jokes mask my tears
A cheerful nature the void

In my soul, my body
Bones shattering
The slivers tearing away
At my spirit
My self esteem
Hating myself for giving in

I break down
Begging for someone to believe
My tears finally free
As someone understands
And takes me in hand
Finally the help I need
My future may yet hold light

I spent that week at home. I had to miss a midterm in organic chemistry. I was not going to classes. My professors were all very understanding; they had seen me struggling around campus with the cane and so they knew something was going on. The Morphine made me violently sick. I remember at some point, after eating a salad, I threw up in the sink because it was too painful to kneel. I had to stand there and scoop up the chunks of lettuce and other vegetables by hand from the sink and throw them into the toilet. Despite being strong enough to make me dizzy and nauseated, the pills barely took the edge off my pain. It was as though I hadn't taken anything. I felt as though my leg didn't actually work. Every step was a matter of supporting my entire weight on the cane until I could inch my back leg past my front leg.

During this time, my parents sent me a care package that I had been requesting for months. The day after I received it, I got a call from the doctor at the hospital I had gone to last. Despite his best efforts, the earliest he could get me an MRI was a month later. The prospect of the future loomed before my eyes. For the next month I would be stuck, unable to move, sick, eating whatever food I could manage to have delivered. I knew I couldn't do it. In despair, I called my parents.

While we had lived in Saskatoon, my parents were actively involved in the Polish community. We had made many friends, and many of them were doctors. When we moved to St. Catharines, a fairly large number of those doctor friends had either already moved to the surrounding areas, or did so within a few years, thus my family had connections within the medical community in the Niagara region. While my parents were aware throughout this process about what was going on with me, I had not previously considered the possibility of going home. I wanted to handle it on my own. I wanted to show that I was a capable adult and that I could take care of myself. This was my second year living on my own, and I wanted that independence. I craved it. My parents, for all that they will deny it, are very controlling. Going home would mean admitting I had failed, and for me, that is a very difficult thing to accept.

I called my parents and told them that I was desperate. I couldn't take another month of this. I needed help. Within an hour, I had a plane ticket back to St. Catharines.

My flatmates, Heather and Andrew, who had been very helpful throughout this process, helped me pack my suitcase. They accompanied me to the airport in a cab. Heather quickly grabbed a wheelchair, and while one of them wheeled me to the counter, another one helped carry my bags. Andrew even received special permission to wheel me through security and wait with me on the other side.

Going through the airport in a wheelchair is a different experience than going through with a cane. With a cane, you have to hobble through while they scan the piece of metal to make sure you aren't concealing anything in the cane. Considering that I usually kept a spare pencil in the pieces of metal, I could understand why they did this. In the past, the security officers had been quite nice. I remember on one occasion, one officer gave me his arm to support me on the way through the metal detector.

When you are in a wheelchair, they know that hobbling is not an option. Instead, you receive a pat down. They run their hands all across the chair to make sure nothing is strapped to it. This would also be my first time flying as someone who needed assistance to get to the plane. When boarding time came, an attendant brought out a special wheelchair, made to take people directly to their seats. They seated me at the front of the plane. When it landed in Toronto, I had to wait for everyone to get off, and then someone came to fetch me. I felt completely helpless.

12 On the Right Track

Within days of getting home, I had an appointment with a rheumatologist, a family friend. She was alarmed by the state I was in. She sent me home with Celebrex, and the promise of an MRI within days. Sure enough, that same week I was getting two MRIs: a plain one and one with barium contrast. In total, I was there for close to two hours, my legs, back, and other limbs supported by pillows in the machine.

When I went back to get the results, most of what she told me came as no surprise. I had a great deal of inflammation and that we would have to treat it aggressively. She started me on chemotherapy, which is used in extreme cases of arthritis to reduce the immune response causing the inflammation. She also gave me a referral to her mentor, a doctor in Toronto who ran a clinic specifically for patients with my type of arthritis.

Treatment would take several months so I had to drop my courses. All the work I had put into my classes were for nothing. If I was able to get better, I would have to repeat the classes again.

The professors were all very helpful. One or two expressed sadness since I had been getting high grades in their class. Still, they knew health was a priority. The university makes you fill out a series of forms to justify dropping out of a semester without penalty on the transcript. We sent in all the forms, filled out by the doctor, along with requests for the science department to forward those same forms to the financial department. The hope was that I might be able to get back my tuition costs for the semester. While my courses were dropped without academic penalty, the forms were never transferred and my tuition was never reimbursed.

The chemo treatment that the doctor started me on was Methotrexate. This medication is known in certain circles as being used to dissolve embryos in ectopic pregnancies. It is also used to treat certain types of cancer and, obviously in my case, autoimmune disorders.

Symptoms I could expect included ulcers, nausea, exhaustion, and bloating, among others. I also had to be on the lookout for more intense symptoms like hair loss, which would mean that I was reacting too strongly to the drug. I took the medication in pill form, eight pills once a week, on Fridays. While on this medication, I could not have any alcohol whatsoever, and it was best if I avoided the sun. Within a few weeks, I came to dread Friday evenings. After taking the meds, I would be out for the night. Feeling weak and sick, I spent much of my time lying down very still so as not to feel worse. Still, the treatment had some effect, and I was able to walk a bit more than I had previously. This is to say my leg was no longer collapsing, and I could drag myself along until I reached some place to sit. I relied heavily on the wheelchairs and mobility-assistance devices that were provided by big stores. Any place that didn't provide any mobility assistive devices became off-limits to me.

The mild improvement in pain levels made it possible for me to leave the house more often, although the side effects of the medication left me fatigued. Before the extreme worsening of my condition, I was able to maintain some semblance of a social life. It helped that while in Ottawa I had met several amazing people who did what they could to spend time with me. In my parent's town, I had fewer friends and little opportunity to meet new people.

Someday

My body screams with the tortures it endures
Chemicals burning through me
Meant to help but also causing more pain
Doubled over as the poisons weave their way
Through my organs taking what they will
Is this really necessary
When Can I be normal again?
Is this what my life will be now?
Saturated with medications
That make me feel worse instead of better
Maybe someday I can live again

Maybe someday I will be free
But for now I endure
In the hopes
Of someday

13 Desperation

It's hard to imagine never-ending pain. Although any given moment we might be hurt, we always assume that, at some point, it will stop. Pain is meant to be a sign that something is wrong, and eventually whatever is wrong is supposed to get better. The virus goes away, the bone heals, the cut scabs over, your hand pulls away from the fire; eventually all the things that cause our pain go away. By this point I had been in near constant pain for months. I felt it even while I slept.

The desperation I had experienced in the previous months was nothing compared to what I felt when I went back to my parents' place. Going back meant failure, plain and simple. It was a big sign saying that I couldn't cut it on my own. I knew that the only way to get my life back was to make the pain go away.

True desperation is a place beyond hope, beyond reason, beyond wanting. It exists as a place of all-consuming need. Everything else is dragged into it like a swirling vortex. I became obsessed with finding some solution for what I was going through. I found endless websites devoted to ways of curing leg pain. Many sites advocated the use of hyperbaric chambers. They claimed that it had something to do with the pressure and the oxygen completely eliminating the inflammation. I started calling around, and soon found a clinic that had such a chamber. It was a holistic medicine clinic that provided a variety of services, everything from orthopedics to naturopathy. I came in for a consultation. The doctor I saw there rejected the idea of the hyperbaric chamber; instead he recommended acupuncture and electrotherapy.

There is a certain level of psychosis associated with severe pain that suggests the strangest solutions for relief; headaches sometimes make you think it's a good idea to bang your head against the wall, joint pain can make you want to crack your joints, and so forth. There is a certain intuitiveness to acupuncture since one of the strange solutions suggested by pain, especially joint pain, is to jab a needle into the part of your body that hurts to help relieve the pressure. The combination of acupuncture and electrotherapy summoned visions of being rigged up like Frankenstein's monsters. Still, it was a possible solution for my pain, so I went for it.

Once a week, I would come into the office to have needles and electrodes placed on my lower back. Although I was desperate for this to work, there was no change other than, perhaps, a slight lessening of pain for the half hour immediately following the appointment.

More effective was the massage I was also getting regularly from a family friend. There are many people who laud massage for its curative powers: if you just get a massage once a week, it will fix your posture, help you grow an inch, improve circulation, cleanse your aura, relieve tension, open your chakras, and all that jazz. Most of that is hokum. What massage will do is help you, and your muscles, relax. When part of your pain is caused by muscular stiffness, this can be a very good thing all on its own. Many autoimmune conditions respond negatively to stress, causing a worsening of symptoms. A massage, through its relaxing atmosphere and release of pressure, is a great way to relieve some of that stress.

While there are benefits to massage, overstating them by incorporating needless mysticism damages its reputation. In an effort to paint massage as something other than a luxury and elevate it into the realm of medical treatment, many practitioners have entered the realm of selling false hopes and snake oil. It says a lot about the world we live in that reducing pain and improving quality of life is considered luxury rather than medicine. That "it makes the patient feel better" is not enough of a positive justification for making something accessible. It shouldn't have to be a miraculous cure to be considered worthwhile.

14 Watch Those Hands, Buddy

Throughout all this time, I was working at my mother's office. Working let me feel less like I was doing nothing, like I was an invalid. I would come in, answer phones, do some editing, and perform other such tasks. One day, my mother came out of her office to let me know that the client inside had seen me walking around with my cane and said he could help me. He was an older man, so both of us assumed that he had some experience with arthritis. Maybe he knew of a new treatment or something that would help take away the pain. I followed her into the room.

The older gentleman smiled at me kindly, and asked me gently if I believed in God. At the time, I still identified as Catholic, though I hadn't been attending church every Sunday in Ottawa. The prospect of getting up early, dragging my pained body onto the bus, and then walking whatever distance to sit on hard, uncomfortable chairs sounded more like torture than salvation. I will talk about religion more in later chapters, but in this context, I want it understood that when I answered yes to his question I was not humoring him. What followed my response almost floored me. The man informed me that he was a faith healer.

Catholics often pride themselves as being less "crazy" than other Christians. They are generally pro-science and pro-medicine, so the idea of faith healing is not one that comes up frequently. Had this happened anywhere else, I probably would have refused his help or laughed it off. In my mother's office however, I didn't feel comfortable doing anything that might upset him. I agreed to let him try to heal me.

My composure was a little harder to keep when he put one hand on my ass and started praying, and soon afterward added his second hand to my crotch. Worse still was when he moving his hands back and forth almost as if he was caressing my ass. I was in shock. I looked up at my mother and then immediately wished I hadn't. The look of shock on her face made me start shaking with suppressed laughter. Soon, I could see my mother also trying to keep in her own chuckles. The man took my shaking as religious ecstasy and continued on with his fervent prayers. By the time he finished, I had tears streaming from my eyes and I felt as though I had fractured a rib from holding in my laughter. I managed to choke out a thank you and headed back to my desk. Once the door was closed and I was safely far enough away, I collapsed with laughter.

At the time the situation seemed something completely out of the ordinary. It wouldn't be till much later that I would learn that abled people feel entitled to the bodies of disabled people. We are often touched against our will, as though we have no agency or bodily autonomy. When this happens, we are expected to smile and be grateful. When paired with the incredibly high rates of sexual assault of people with disabilities, these presumptions become terrifying.

15 Woo

I didn't realize it at the time, but this was just the start of people trying to help me with miracles. Over the course of the next few months, I had people recommend a variety of treatments, frequently involving dietary changes. Some people would insist that the inflammation was a reaction to too much caffeine and that I should give up on tea and coffee. Still others insisted that instead I should look into fish oil. One person's advice often contradicted with another's: eat more iron, eat less iron; all your foods should be cooked, make sure everything you eat is raw; the pain is caused by crystals in your joints, it is all a vitamin D deficiency.

A friend of my parents had equipment in her home that she insisted would help. I didn't know what I was getting into when we went over to her house; I only knew that she had recently started working with some form of "medical" treatments. When we got to her house, there was a mat placed on a table. At first glance, it looked like it might have been a massage bed. I followed instructions and climbed on.

Instead, what followed was an explanation on how inflammation was caused by blood pooling too much in one area. That in order for it to be stopped, the blood needed to be encouraged to flow to other parts of the body. Since blood is made up primarily of iron, you could help encourage this flow by exposing yourself to magnets. The arguments against such assertions are immediately apparent. If your blood was able to respond to magnets in such a way, you could give yourself a bruise with a fridge magnet just by hovering it over your skin. MRIs wouldn't work, since the strong magnetic resonance would quite literally pull the blood out of your body. Still, I didn't want to insult my parents' friend. Sensing my discomfort, she quickly assured me that the magnetic field of the bed was no higher than the magnetic frequency of the earth, that it would safely encourage the pooling blood out of my inflamed joints and back into their "natural flow."

My father, who has some sceptical tendencies of his own, asked how—if the frequency of the bed was the same as that of the earth—using it differed from just lying on a beach somewhere. Apparently it doesn't. In fact, she answered, a beach would be even better since I would also absorb the natural healing rays of the sun. As she continued the explanation, she mentioned how continuing treatments would cost some hundred dollars a session, and buying a bed of my own would cost about a thousand dollars. I think both my dad and I were thinking the same thing: that the money would be better spent on a trip to the beach.

My dad and I must have been joking about something along those lines when we got home because I got a lecture from my mother about keeping an open mind. She told me that I was doing more damage to myself by acting like a little know-it-all. After all, these therapies were being discovered and performed by people who were all older, and thus wiser, than I was. Surely one of them would work.

16 It's All Natural

The idea that alternative medicine is traditional or natural is part of a marketing strategy to legitimize it. The logic assumes that something done for thousands of years must surely have some benefit. The argument is disingenuous since most cultures today reject many things that were once traditional, such as arranged marriage and slavery. Why, if we have abandoned other traditions, do we so desperately cling to antiquity as a sign of efficacy?

It is much the same with the concept of "natural." I've had these conversations before in coffee shops: someone trying to convince me that natural is so much better, all the while gorging themselves on their soy milk latte and cake made with fresh berries, in the middle of winter in Canada. Humans have spent thousands of years defying nature to improve our lives, yet we still seem to think that the "natural" label on our herbal supplements is a guarantee that they will be safe and effective. To judge medication by the standard of natural or unnatural is meaningless for several reasons, one of the most obvious being that many of the pharmaceuticals seen as unnatural are merely the results of improvements to old herbal remedies.

Take willow bark tea and aspirin for example. At some point in our history, people noticed that if you made a tea from the bark of a willow tree, you could reduce fevers and swelling. True, you would have a horrible stomach ache afterward, and if you drank too much of it you would end up vomiting blood, but it was still a revolutionary discovery. Years later, scientists identified the chemical in willow bark tea that has these amazing properties. They called it acetylsalicylic acid (ASA). They then combined it with stomach guards to prevent the ulcers caused by the tea and called it aspirin.

So can herbal treatments work? Yes, they can, but they are dangerous. You see, it's harder to standardize potency in an herbal treatment. How much of the useful ingredient a plant contains depends on many factors: the quality of the herb, when in its life cycle it was harvested, even the time of day that it was harvested, how long it was sitting around before being used, the temperature at which it was distilled, and so forth. If herbalists took the time to control for all those factors, they would be creating pharmaceutical drugs, and not herbal treatments.

What's more, the contents of herbal treatments can be unreliable too. There have been multiple situations in which the wrong herb was accidentally substituted for the one intended, sometimes with deadly results. The mechanical harvesting techniques employed by many big herbal companies, or a simple lack of attention, could mean that the herbal treatment is contaminated with weeds or other invasive plants unknowingly harvested at the same time. There are fewer controls in place to make sure that what is written on the bottle matches what is in the capsule.

What pharmacologists, chemists, and pharmacists do is isolate what is useful and dispose of the rest. They adjust for safe and effective dosage. They have to meet strident standards of purity, effectiveness, safety, etc. When a bottle of aspirin says that a capsule contains 250mg of ASA, they mean it. It doesn't mean that it contains X amount of willow bark that, if conditions are optimal, should contain 250mg of ASA. No, each capsule will contain exactly 250mg of ASA. Not only that, but they can tell you exactly how much is safe to take and how much you need to take for it to work. Pharmaceuticals are nature perfected for maximum benefit and minimum risk.

There are two primary targets for predatory promoters of alternative medication: the patient and the patient's family. In both cases, they rely on the fear that comes from uncertainty. When you are dealing with pain, whether or not you know the cause, you and those around you are suffering as much from not knowing how to stop it as you are from experiencing it. The unknown can be so strong that, once you have an explanation of why you are sick or in pain, your symptoms can dramatically improve on their own. Many people also report that just going to the doctor and knowing they are going to be helped can make them feel better. Complementary and alternative medicine (CAM) practitioners who provide pseudo medical services know it works this way. There is no need for whatever they are peddling to actually work, because just making it seem like they have the answer will do most of their work for them. The rest can be taken care of through the placebo effect.

Patients suffer from the desperation that comes from actually being sick or in pain. Family and friends, on the other hand, suffer the desperation that comes from not being able to do anything to help. They feel useless and, in that uselessness, they desperately search for something that they can do to make everything better for their loved ones. Enter the CAM practitioner.

Real medicine is a testament to human accomplishment. Alternative medicine, however, presents itself as being on the one hand a discipline of knowledge, but on the other hand accessible to anyone. The layperson assumes that naturopaths, homeopaths, and other such practitioners have as much study behind them as doctors. On the surface at least, the "knowledge" they are peddling is usually comprehensible and makes some intuitive sense. The friend or family member stumbles across this arcane bit of knowledge, and they pass it on, feeling as though they are helping. In some cases, they might go so far as to force the patient to participate so that they can feel as though they are contributing to their long-term rehabilitation. When the patient fails to get better, the fear turns into anger. By not getting better, the patient is demonstrating their lack of commitment, which in turn means a lack of gratitude for the knowledge they have been given.

While CAM practitioners succeed by showing glimpses of improvement and hope, they require fear to sell their products and treatments. Fear clouds judgment, it clouds scepticism. Fear is the grandparent of irrationality.

There is a tendency among skeptic communities to mock users of alternative medicine as being unintelligent. It is, however, not a matter of intelligence. Rather, it is a matter of distraction caused by fear. The most intelligent person in the world can be tricked if caught at the right time. Educating people about the dangers of alternative therapies is important, but in order for this education to be effective, it has to start before the person is even a patient. Even then, however, it might not work if the person is overwhelmed enough, willing to try anything that offers even the possibility of hope. Rather, in order to stop the preying tendency of pseudoscience, we must create a community that demands evidence and fosters critical thinking at every level. We must encourage comprehensive science education that is accessible for all, and we must impose the same strict standards of effectiveness on all forms of treatment as are placed on true medicine. Beyond even that, we must create communities that work toward lessening desperation in patients and their families, through community outreach and through research into effective treatments for a variety of ailments.

Doctors themselves are harming their reputation when they maintain attitudes of superiority. Many patients abandoned modern medicine in favor of alternative therapies because the medical establishment failed them first. That failure is often the result of arrogance and unwillingness to listen to patients. Sometimes, it's beyond the doctors' control, such as when they are strained by inefficient healthcare systems. The inability to listen to a patient is fostered as much by attitude as by the waiting rooms filled to bursting because there are not enough family doctors and nurse practitioners to meet the needs of our communities. When you add to that the financial barriers that exist in places that do not have socialized medicine, you create a system that is overwhelmed and unable to meet the needs of its populace.

I never did go back for another session on the magnetic bed. There was no point.

17 Depression

Since returning home, I had spent all my free time reading or watching TV. I had made no effort to get out of my parents' house or to reconnect with the people I knew in the area. I didn't know it at the time, but these were the first symptoms of the depression that my extended suffering had pushed me into.

There is this misconception that depression is about sadness, that it is just what happens when someone is very sad and can't get over it. While I won't speak for everyone, for me depression was not so much sadness but a lack of energy. It was almost like extreme burnout. I was neither happy nor sad; I was just unable to muster up the energy to do anything or feel anything.

I mentioned previously that, in coming home, I felt as though I had failed. Well, since I had already failed, this meant I didn't have to try anymore. The only light at the end of the tunnel was the idea that, someday, the pain would end and I could build myself up again.

Chronic illnesses like arthritis, Crohn's, lupus, and many others often go hand in hand with depression. It is the feeling of uselessness that accompanies being sick. When you are too tired to do anything, when you need to rely on other people just to get by, you feel as though you have no purpose. Everyone else seems to be contributing something to the world at large, but you, the sick person, don't see any contribution of your own. Dragging yourself out of bed is a chore, and so you sink into the feeling that there is no point in leaving it. My life seemed to stretch out endlessly before me, never ending, and never changing.

My depression manifested itself as a feeling of numbness. The kind of numbness that come not from an absence of pain but from being so swamped and overwhelmed by it that I just couldn't feel anymore. Not just physical pain, but also the overwhelming emotional pain that accompanies it. You stop feeling at all as a form of self-preservation. The problem, of course, is that not doing anything doesn't restore your energy; it actually drains it even more. The longer you lie in bed, the harder it becomes to leave it. But alternatives were hard to consider when it hurt so much just to move or get up.

At some point discussions came up in my family about the long term. It seemed that the most likely scenarios were that I would end up needing surgery, biologics (medications that modulate the immune system), or both. Any option meant that the likelihood of me going back to Ottawa was rapidly diminishing. My parents spent a significant amount of time trying to convince me that I would be better off staying at home in St. Catharines, where they could take care of me and keep an eye on me. The more they discussed that possibility, the more I began considering the possibility of ending my life.

For all that I love my family, our relationship is adversarial at best. Being home always meant putting on more weight, heightening anxiety, and desperately hiding as much of the real me as possible. My mother, who is convinced that I am a compulsive liar, doesn't realize that hiding the truth from them is a matter of survival. Throughout high school, my mantra was *just four more years till I can move away to university, just three more years, just two more years, just one more year, just six more months, just two more weeks, just one more night, just five more minutes . . .* The prospect of coming back permanently was one I couldn't face. I knew that if a time came when my options ran out and I would be stuck there, that would be the moment that I would end my life.

Depression is often represented as selfishness and weakness. This image adds to the feeling of self-loathing that already goes hand in hand. It encourages people to hide what they are feeling and experiencing, which in turn increases the feelings of loneliness. It is a desperate cycle that ends in either trusting someone and getting help or in tragedy.

There is a new trend on Facebook and other social media sites that talk about depression in more positive terms. Posts that talk about the strength it takes to live with depression, anxiety, and similar disabilities. Some claim that these types of statements glorify mental illness, that they make it seem like it's okay to be depressed. Such people may claim that *real* strength comes from seeking help, rather than "wallowing" in self-pity. What people like that fail to understand is that the world is already working to make anyone with a mental illness feel like they are worthless, and that seeking help can be great but that it is not always an option for everyone.

In my case, talking to someone was out of the question. I had no one nearby who I could ask for help, and reaching out to my family would be tantamount to declaring war. Sometime after I had returned to live with my parents, I remember my mother making a big deal about how offended she was that it took me as long to come home as it did. It was all about her, and she insisted that my not coming to her at the first twinge was nothing more than a slap in her face. I was an ungrateful child who didn't appreciate everything that she had done for me. When I pointed out how she had always disregarded my joint pain in the past, the whole situation blew up. I ended up having to grovel for forgiveness as every bad thing I have ever done was brought up.

Imagine telling them that the thought of being forced to remain home was making me suicidal. Being at home meant that I was forced to interact constantly with the people who were directly responsible for my anxiety issues. It is not an exaggeration when I say that I exhibit symptoms of PTSD before every trip home.

18 Faith

I was often recommended to go talk to a religious leader, like a priest. If I could only find God, I was told, all my bad feelings would go away. It is my experience, however, that religious leaders are among the worst choice for help when it comes to any form of mental illness. Catholicism, for example, is very harsh about suicide. The belief is that if you kill yourself, you will end up immediately in hell. These beliefs about the eternal consequences of suicide also translate into a negative stigma surrounding those who reach that point. God can help pull you out of depression, but being depressed in the first place must mean you weren't devout enough already.

In reality, churches have little motivation to fight depression since it helps them thrive. In much of North American society, we are taught from a young age that, if you are desperate, you should seek solace in the ever-open, ever-loving arms of an almighty deity. The teaching that God, however you might imagine that concept, loves you no matter what can provide momentary relief in depression. The sense of community and belonging that many feel when going to church also helps. Then there's the routine; going to church means having to get up, to clean yourself, and to interact with other people. All of those actions can provide a temporary relief from many of the feelings that come with depression.

But rather than recognizing that the positive effects stem from getting out of the house, seeing other people, and taking a shower for the first time in who knows how long, people attribute any improvement to divine healing. Ultimately, however, you crash as the feelings of inadequacy come back. You haven't actually done anything to actually help your depression; you just found temporary respite. For those who believe that their reprieve was the work of a deity, they may then start suffering from a sense of divine abandonment once their overwhelming feelings return. The lord has forsaken you, and you must therefore be unworthy of help.

This self-perpetuating cycle is difficult to break out of as church attendance and religious observance become associated with a sense of improvement, but the lack of any real improvement solidifies the grasp of your disease on you. The more depressed you become, the more you feel that you need the church, but the more you go to church, the more depressed you become. The ultimate result is your unhappiness while the church thrives. It is only when things reach a terminal level, when you commit suicide, that your benefit to the church disappears.

The fact that I was thinking about suicide at all would paint me as weak. I would be instructed to put my faith in God and to stop being selfish. The advice would undermine any self-confidence that remained in me. It would increase my social isolation as I wondered who in the parish now knew. Moreover, eventually, it would get back to my family and I would be in the same circumstance as always.

Normally in such a situation, the best place to seek help would be from the medical community. The fear here, however, was that I was already having enough trouble trying to get help for my hip. If I added to it the possibility of a psychological disorder, the likelihood of being taken seriously would disappear even more. I would lose what progress I had made and would once again be relegated to the status of drug seeker. There were already many people who insisted that the pain was all in my head. I was scared to give voice to the problems that really were in my head, lest the physical symptoms that landed me in that state be once again ignored as a product of my imagination.

I had no one to confide in. My friends were all back in Ottawa, and it seemed I had left my life there as well. What ultimately helped was eventually being able to talk myself out of the house to reconnect with an old friend. He was in a wheelchair, and his example helped give me the perspective I needed to deal with my own loss of mobility.

19 Vacation Woes

While we waited for the appointment with the specialist, my parents decided to go on a family vacation to Cuba. We had gone before. I imagined lying poolside reading, enjoying nice swims, and eating great food. I was excited. What I didn't realize was the extent to which chemo and sun don't mix.

My lack of mobility made it hard to apply the sunscreen before going out. I had to rely on spray creams, which often left the floor treacherously slippery. Swimming was more pleasant than walking, but the direct sunlight left me feeling nauseated and weak.

Our cabana was on the opposite end of the resort from the restaurants. If I wanted to have dinner, I had to arrange for transport to take me from my room all the way there. In a short time, I realized there was little point in leaving my room. Despite being one of the best resorts I had been to, I spent the majority of my time in my room with the blinds drawn. My day was spent watching TV and reading. My parents would bring me food from the restaurants, which I occasionally supplemented with room service.

One night, after managing to leave the room for a little bit, I came back to find a bug the size of my palm on the bed. I shrieked, and my dad came in and got rid of it. Apparently, it had been attracted by the food in the room.

Although a trip of that sort was a luxury that I really appreciated, especially in light of my own inability to afford it, between my pains and the nausea from the chemo, it is one that would have been best avoided.

Looking back it was a harsh reminder that most resorts don't cater to those with disabilities. It is not all that surprising when one considers the links between poverty and disability, but it is a harsh reminder that here to is another world that is inaccessible for those who are different.

20 The Specialist

Eventually my appointment with the specialist in Toronto arrived. Before I saw her, she sent in one of her students to ask questions, take mobility measurements, and gather information for her to make her assessment. After answering, I sat waiting in the room with my father.

At this first meeting, the doctor burst into the room looking at my chart and talking about surgery before even looking up at me. I felt as though I was caught in a whirlwind. After months of inactivity, all of a sudden everything was happening so fast. No having to try and explain myself, no trying to force her to look past my age, this doctor knew I was there because it was serious, and she was acting like it. She wanted to have the surgery done as soon as possible. Within moments, I was having an X-ray to get the latest look at my hip

After the imaging was done, we were able to slow down. There was still a chance to avoid surgery. While the damage was bad, and showed significant neglect on the part of other doctors, there was still some cartilage left in my joints. It would never grow back, but if we could stop the inflammation, I could avoid needing surgery for a while. There was time, but not a lot of it. If I had had to wait even two more weeks, too much damage might have been done and a hip replacement would have been unavoidable. The doctor told me that she was shocked that I was still walking at all. According to her, with that level of inflammation, most others would have lost consciousness from pain had they attempted to walk. Here I was, despite the pain, dragging myself around with a cane.

Her recommendation was Enbrel—the very medication that had been recommended by my family friend months prior at the Christmas party. I didn't make the connection at the time of the appointment. Later I felt so angry that I had had the answer so early and had it denied to me.

Enbrel works by inhibiting an antibody known as tumor necrosis factor. While I was on it, I would be highly susceptible to upper respiratory infections. Moreover, my risks of lymphoma in the long run would double. A new drug still under patent, it would be expensive. She explained the procedure for getting on Trillium, a provincial prescription drug coverage program, and the process for getting government approval for the drug. It would be important for me to get a tuberculosis test done, since that infection in particular was dangerous for me. In order to save my hip from surgery, it was important that I start the medication as soon as possible. One thing my parents have always been generous with, to their credit, is their money. They agreed to pay for the medication out of pocket until the needed coverage could be arranged. Had that not been possible, I likely would be sporting an implant now.

I quickly arranged to have the tests done, and within a short period of time, I had a nurse at my home explaining how to administer the drug. I would have to inject myself once a week, in my thigh. The use of an auto-injector meant that I would never have to see the needle as it was going in. The whole process was relatively smooth, and while I certainly didn't look forward to the injections, it was still a great improvement to what had been going on previously.

Within days, I was walking more surely. I was still a little stiff and sore at first but the improvement was dramatic. We went to Pelee Island just two weeks later, and it was on this trip that I was able to summon the strength to ride a bike. Soon, I was able to abandon the cane altogether. I was better, and all I had to do was inject myself once a week.

One of the best rewards was that I returned to Ottawa and moved into a new apartment. I wasn't able to walk as far or as fast as I had before, and I got tired or sore faster, but I felt better than I had in months. I felt like I was independent again.

I did my best to get my life back to normal. I was still on chemo, which meant I wasn't allowed to consume any alcohol, but I got a boyfriend and life seemed to be moving in the right direction. It wasn't that long before I became sexually active and discovered that sex was a great form of physiotherapy. No other form of exercise did nearly as much to help regain some bit of mobility in my right hip.

My introduction to sex was somewhat less than glamorous, but had the side benefit of making for a great story. We were watching *The Lord of the Rings* together and started fooling around. I decided that I was ready to "do the deed," and let him know.

After a mad scramble to pick up some condoms at the gas station across the street, we quickly got back to his apartment. Just as he was about to enter me for the first time I noticed the movie was still on, right at the scene where Gandalf faces the Balrog. The words that accompanied my loss of virginity were "You Shall Not Pass!"

I thought I would die, or at least crack a rib, from the strain of trying to keep from laughing. Probably not the sentiment the guy was hoping for at the time. It didn't help that our first kiss also had me breaking out in a fit of giggles, thrown off balance as I was by the taste of cigarette ash.

Eventually I was told I could wean myself off Methotrexate, the chemo drug I had been on. The Enbrel had no side effects I was aware of. There were still things I couldn't do: my hip clicked whenever I rode a bike, and I was expressly forbidden by doctors to run. My mobility was improving slightly, but I still couldn't bend enough to tie my right shoe— something I am still unable to do. Bending over in general causes difficulty and pain.

Part 2: Crohn's Disease

21 A Bit of a Pain in the Behind

My boyfriend and I broke up and I met someone else, someone more suited to me. Within the first few weeks of us dating, I developed intense stomach pain and went to the ER. I was put on an IV and they gave me painkillers while they ran tests. The drugs they gave me had the curious side effect of making me think the walls were melting. I watched the clock stretch out as it slid down the walls. The paint was sliding off like spilled molasses, as was each subsequent coat: hospital gown green, pink, yellowish beige, each revealing itself one by one.

I was worried that it was a resurgence of the pancreatitis I had had a few years before.

Over the next eighteen hours, I had blood drawn for a multitude of tests as they tested me for everything that made sense: appendicitis, infection, and other such considerations. I was asked to stay in the hospital overnight, until the ultrasound clinic opened the next morning. My new boyfriend spent the entire night with me, and we took turns trying to catch what sleep we could on the hard examination table. This was before the hospital rooms came equipped with beds. After the ultrasound, when no clear cause presented itself, they simply sent me home. There was some mention of a colonoscopy, and I was told that they would call me.

Eventually the pain went away and I forgot about it. I focused on school and the interesting classes I was taking. Sometime during the semester, I found a lump in the space between my bum and my thigh. This wasn't an unusual occurrence; throughout puberty I was blessed with few blemishes on my face, but I would get little lumps along the crease between my genitals and my leg instead. They would be hard and painful, but eventually I would pop them and they would go away, just like any other pimple. When I found this lump, I figured it would be no different.

I was slightly disturbed by its size, though, which was bigger than most other blemishes I had had. Also, it was a lot more difficult to pop. It had never taken me more than a day or two to wear away at it enough to squeeze out. This one, however, proved difficult and resisted most of my efforts, and it was some weeks later when I managed to pop it. By this point the lump had become very painful and the release of pressure did a lot to help alleviate that. Strangely, this was not the end of it. Within a few hours, the lump seemed to refill with the same greenish pus that had flowed out previously. I spent some time doing what I could to empty it again.

Over the next week or two, I had a strange routine. I would empty the lump, then, after a while, I would develop a sharp pain that would radiate out from the area of the lump. This would prompt me to go to the washroom and drain it again. When I was able to find some time, I finally went to a clinic to get the thing checked out. The doctor who saw me explained that it was an abscess. With the help of some towels, she tried to completely empty it and then prescribed me some antibiotics. The inflammation around the abscess went down, and it was no longer filling with fluid to the same extent, but the thing itself did not go away. I went back to the doctor and she sent me a referral to a surgeon.

Since it was no longer infected and most of the pain was gone, the appointment was scheduled for some weeks later. In the meantime, I started a job at a men's clothing store. Work was pretty fun, though from time to time I would be seized by a stomach cramp that had me bending over in pain. The sudden cramps lasted for a short time and were promptly forgotten. I assumed that my more active lifestyle was just causing gas pains.

My meeting with the surgeon was short. He took a quick look and told me that the abscess was no longer an abscess and had become a fistula: a connection between two organs that normally don't have a connection. In this case, it was a connection between my anal glands and my skin. I would need outpatient surgery where they would cut it open and let it seal as it healed. The surgery was scheduled for a few weeks later.

In the meantime, I continued working. I didn't notice at the time that I was rapidly losing weight. I had always gone to the bathroom frequently, but it had been recently increasing—I would have as many as eight loose bowel movements a day. I didn't really pay attention to that either, though, since it didn't seem to be causing any problems. I had heard about irritable bowel syndrome and figured that was the problem. I did not connect the frequent bathroom trips with the occasional stomach cramps.

22 I Have What?!

I had been combining my appointments with the specialist in Toronto with short visits to my family. While I was there, my mother remarked that I seemed to be going to the bathroom more frequently. She bugged me about it, and I told her that it was nothing. That I probably just had irritable bowels, which I had heard was common with arthritis. Since it wasn't bothering me, I argued, what was the problem?

In truth, my frequent bathroom trips—while annoying—didn't displease me. I was sure they were a sign of my increasing metabolism and were in part responsible for my weight, which had been a concern, moving in the right direction. I, uncharitably, wrote off my mother's concern as jealousy over my weight loss, and anger that she no longer had it to use against me.

A few weeks before I was scheduled for surgery, I flew down for the weekend to St. Catharines. While I was there, I had a follow-up appointment with the specialist in Toronto. The doctor was pleased with my progress, and confided in me that it almost seemed as though the impossible was happening and some of my cartilage was regenerating. We discussed the possibility of referring me to one of her colleagues in Ottawa who would be able to follow me from that point on.

I brought up my upcoming surgery to find out how long I would need to be off Enbrel. What followed was so unexpected that I could barely move as my doctor burst out angrily, yelling, "Why didn't you tell me you had Crohn's disease?" I sat there in shock while she raged about the fact that I would skew her results and make it seem as though Enbrel caused the disorder. When I got back to the car with my dad, I burst out crying.

At this point in time, I had only ever heard of Crohn's once. I had no idea what it did, I had only heard a friend mention a past boyfriend who had it and spent the majority of his life in the hospital, in extreme pain, and on horrible drugs. I had had no idea that anything else was wrong with me or that the fistula could be the symptom of something else. I was on the verge of hysteria. My dad decided to call a friend who was a nurse for her husband, a renowned gynecologist in our region. With luck she would know something and be able to give us some quick advice.

She explained that there are many people with Crohn's in the Polish-Canadian community, and that it wasn't the death sentence I had initially thought it would be. I can't remember much of what she said, but whatever it was, it was enough to help me calm down and push the doctor's words from my mind.

23 Surgery

I went off the Enbrel in preparation for the upcoming surgery. I had some concerns about the leg pain coming back, so I confided to my boss that I might have some slight difficulty with my legs during that time.

About two weeks before the surgery was scheduled, I started feeling really ill. I was overwhelmed with nausea and the intermittent cramps I had been experiencing got stronger. I was worried about any complications this could cause during the surgery, so I went to the hospital. They did a quick onceover and mentioned that I might have a mild liver infection. They sent me home with some antibiotics.

Coming home and thinking about it, I considered the possibility that all this was the result of my birth control. I knew from the warnings on the inserts in the packages that hormonal contraceptives could occasionally cause liver issues. Since I was receiving frequent blood tests related to my leg issue, I wasn't getting expressly tested for liver issues associated with the birth control as often as was recommended. I had a discussion with my boyfriend, and I decided to go off the contraceptives for a short period of time to see if that helped with the issues I had been having.

The day of the surgery arrived. When the anaesthesiologist came in, I warned him that I had a tendency to metabolize medications very quickly. He informed me that they would either be sedating me or, if need be, putting me under. Putting me under would require them to put a tube in my throat. After my experience getting an endoscopy, this concerned me. Still, I trusted them to do what needed doing. On the operating table, I fell promptly asleep.

I came to as I heard someone say, "Okay, we're done here." I drowsily responded with "We're done?"

I heard the sound of clattering instruments and expletives, and someone asking me if I was really awake. If I was, it didn't last long as the doctor lunged from where he was standing to push more sedation and put me back to sleep. I woke up quite a while later. As soon as I woke, I needed to have a bowel movement. This surprised the nurses as I had had to clear myself out for the surgery, so there should not have been anything left to pass.

I was given some Tylenol with codeine and sent home. The pain was manageable, and I didn't feel like I needed the painkillers. The next morning my postcare nurse arrived. As part of the healing process, the wound had to be packed with gauze to make sure that it healed in the right direction. If it healed from the outside in, I ran the risk of infection and another abscess. The process of packing was brutal. It was essentially using a blunt toothpick to push gauze into a fresh cut. I cried out, to the point where I woke my roommate and apparently terrified him as well.

This torture would have to be repeated regularly for close to two weeks. The concentrated pain in that area seemed to stimulate my need to go to the washroom. This was a relatively new pattern that I had started to notice: whenever I felt a twinge of pain, I would have to go to the bathroom almost immediately. I would go to the washroom, and the process would push out the packed gauze. It felt like I was putting up with the pain for nothing.

24 Food Poisoning

In the days after my surgery, my mornings involved visits from the nurse and the packing of my incision, and the rest of the day remained relatively calm and straightforward. I took frequent warm baths after each trip to the bathroom. At some point, my flatmates and I noticed that we were all starting to feel a little ill. I had started throwing up again, and many of the others were looking green about the gills. We discovered that our fridge was broken and not cooling our food sufficiently. We all had food poisoning.

When we asked our property manager to fix the issue, we were told that it would be two weeks before we could get a new fridge. We were told this after we had already waited a week and a half for a response. Finally, I managed to convince our property manager to agree to pay half the costs for us to get a deep freezer.

We all felt better within a few days, but I was soon sick again. I figured that I had just come down with the flu or a cold, that I was just unlucky. The fact that I had a mild fever seemed to confirm my assumption. I started feeling cold all the time. Even though it was the middle of summer, I was constantly shivering. At work, especially, I would be really cold. Finally, after a whole week of barely being able to keep even liquids down, I went to the hospital. They put me on an IV to boost up my fluids and, after a few hours, sent me home.

Getting the fluids helped me feel better for a few days, but then I started getting sick again. It got to the point where I was constantly nauseated and I was spending a night at the hospital every few days. I would get an IV, an ultrasound, and be sent home with the instructions that I needed a colonoscopy.

No matter how often I was told I needed one, however, they never seemed to arrange for one. Whenever I asked, I was told they would call me with an appointment soon, but none ever seemed to be forthcoming.

In the back of my mind, whispered so quietly that I could pretend I didn't hear it, were the arthritis specialist's words: Crohn's. Still, I didn't want to believe it.

On one hospital visit, I was concerned by the pain that had started accompanying my nausea more and more frequently. I started to worry that I had an ulcer. Though I wasn't throwing up blood, I felt like I could taste it in the back of my throat. One of the nurses took me aside as they discharged me, and told me that if the pain was bothering me, she could give me a recipe for the "poor man's morphine." All I had to do, she said, was take four extra strength Tylenols and three Advil. I was floored. Here I was worried about an ulcer, and this woman was giving me a prescription to make sure I would be in bringing up blood in a matter of hours. I worried about the other people she might have been hurting. Not many people know this, but NSAIDS like Advil, Aleve, aspirin, and others irritate the stomach and make ulcers more likely. Many don't realize that NSAIDs should always be taken with food, or at least a glass of something to drink, to help ease the impact.

Around this time, one of my ankles also started hurting. I had a tendency to roll my feet pretty often, so I assumed that I had twisted something. When the other one started hurting, I worried that my arthritis had moved on to a new joint. By this point I had not restarted my Enbrel, waiting for the go-ahead from my doctors. With biologics, you want to make sure that you don't take them when you are sick. Since they act as immunosuppressants, it can increase the risk of infection and make sickness last longer.

I was soon walking with my cane again, this time using it almost like a crutch to help with my ankles.

At some point, I weighed myself and realized that I had lost over thirty pounds in one month. I knew I was in trouble. Not prepared to go through the same hurdles I'd had to go through to have my leg taken seriously, I called my parents and asked them to arrange for me to come back to St. Catharines for a bit.

By this point my ankles had both swollen and looked as though they had baseballs attached to them. The pain was different from what my arthritis usually felt like, more like pins and needles. I kept both ankles wrapped up as though they were sprained.

Between the pain in my ankles, the pain in my guts, and feeling weak from being unable to keep any food down, I could do almost nothing while there. I spent most of my day lying in bed reading or on the computer. Despite the trouble I've had with my mother, I do have to take a moment to point out when the situation is dire she is in her element.

I am grateful for the time she spent massaging soothing oil into my ankles to help the swelling go down and help take some of the pain away. She would also bring me soothing beverages and prepare easy to digest foods. I feel that she is never as happy as when she has someone relying on her completely. In those moments, she is everything you could want in a mother: warm, caring, and compassionate. As long as she gets to be completely in control, and completely needed, she is happy.

When things improve under her care, however, she goes back to her old tricks. When I was able to hobble around again, she began to lecture me on how she always knew that there was something seriously wrong with me, and if I had just listened to her months earlier, everything would have been fine. While there is an element of truth to that statement, what it ignores is the fact that her worries were somehow nonexistent back in high school and elementary school when I expressed concerns about the pain in my joints and the frequent stomach aches I had. The many hours where I would cry that certain foods made me sick. Instead when I asked to see the doctor I was told I was just a picky eater, too fat, and too much of a hypochondriac. That it was all in my head. But now all I heard was how she always knew there was something wrong with me. History has a way of rewriting itself with the addition of hindsight.

The day after arriving in St. Catharines, I was sitting in my family doctor's office, seeing one of his associates. The swelling in my joints, and whatever was going on with my digestive issue, were immediately linked. I was given prednisone, a steroid often used to treat flares of autoimmune conditions and told once again that I needed a colonoscopy.

Despite hearing for over a year that it was something I needed, the hospital had still not contacted me about an appointment. There is a lot of talk about the long wait times for tests in Canada. Many people tout it as a failure of socialized medicine. The assumption is that the system is clogged up with unnecessary tests being run by worried hypochondriacs. In actuality the timing of tests are organized according to urgency, with each level being assigned a certain number of regular spots. Emergency cases take priority over others as they are needed to determine immediate life or death situations. For example, in the case of colonoscopies, one might be needed for someone passing significant blood, where the source of the leak needs to be isolated. Urgent cases include patients admitted to the hospital or those who need the test prior to leaving the hospital. Then there are the semiurgent cases where an answer is required soon, but the patient is able to wait at home in the meantime. Finally there are the regularly scheduled cases, which receive a certain number of spaces each month so as not to be completely overwhelmed by the more pressing cases.

What often ends up happening is that emergency and regular cases get scheduled within a reasonable period of time, while the urgent and semiurgent cases compete for spaces. Since patients admitted in the hospital take priority, it is the semi-urgent cases that often find themselves as the ones waiting the longest, or so it appears. This is information I've gathered as someone who has occupied each of these levels of urgency.

Since I had to this point never been formally admitted into the hospital, the scheduling for my tests was deemed a lesser priority. By this point in my story, I had not yet had an appointment scheduled.

Now, however, the level of urgency had increased. I was becoming an emergency case and ranked high on the urgency scale. St. Catharines has the added advantage of also being a smaller city, and so the overall wait time was shorter to being with. My family doctor managed to schedule an appointment two weeks from my visit.

By this point, my frequent bathroom trips were starting to get to me. I felt as though my skin was rubbed raw. When I went back for a precolonoscopy examination a few days later, my doctor had to insert his finger into my anus. I was so swollen that even though he used only his smallest finger, I felt as if I was being torn apart.

I started doing research into irritable bowel disorders. I discovered that many of them could cause joint swelling, which would explain what was going on with my foot. I convinced myself that the most likely answer was ulcerative colitis, burying my thoughts of Crohn's disease.

My appointment for the colonoscopy arrived quite quickly. I had had to stop the prednisone a week or more before to make sure it didn't mask what was wrong with me. I needn't have bothered. My intestines were so swollen that the doctor was afraid to go very high. He told me I would have to get an appointment with a gastroenterologist (or GI doctor) and wait for the biopsy results, but that it seemed likely that I had ulcerative colitis.

25 Mixed Messages

During this time, I received strange mixed messages. Many people told me that I didn't look sick. Some would say things along the lines of "I know you are sick, but you look fantastic!" I was irritated by those comments. While I didn't have an eating disorder, the visible effects mimicked bulimia quite closely. The compliments I received just reinforced this idea that if I ever did become bulimic, the members of my church and community would be on board. After all, it doesn't matter what you feel like, it's appearance that is important.

We are so obsessed with outward appearance in our culture, that the goal of looking our best sometimes supersedes every other facet of our lives. It is why people are willing to try out lifestyle changes that make themselves miserable in order to achieve some arbitrary (and unattainable) standard of physical attractiveness.

There is this belief that if you can make yourself beautiful, that you will be happy. The horrible irony of the situation of course is that the pursuit of that goal often makes you miserable. It is not surprising that this is the case, when our society puts such pressure on everyone to fall within a very constrictive standard. If we diversified the concept of attractiveness and beauty, how many people would really be willing to put up with the juice cleanses, the restrictive diets, and the various other ways people strive to achieve that standard.

It is a symptom of the messed-up social cues surrounding appearance, especially in women. Despite the fact that my life was draining away, what was important was that I was losing weight. I've actually heard people console those going on chemo or other horrible treatments by saying, "Well, at least it will help you lose weight."

In an attempt to help people "think positive" about their illness, often people try to point out supposed benefits. "I wish I could sleep all day!" "You're so skinny!" "Now you get to smoke pot whenever you want. You're so lucky!" The intent is a good one, but the result ends up being dehumanizing, and enraging. I sleep all day because I don't have the energy to get up, even if I want to. I am skinny because my body is slowly starving to death. I smoke pot because I am in constant pain or always feel nauseated. The supposed benefits of our illnesses are actually either direct symptoms or meant to make our lives less terrible. The things that are great in small doses are actually excruciating when forced on you.

By bringing up these supposed benefits as positives, the person speaking is ignoring the lived experience of the other person in order to feel less terrible about what is going on. Sick people are downers, but if we can come up with reasons why what they are going through isn't that bad, then we don't have to spend time thinking about things that make us sad. The consequence of this is that by sugar coating what is going on, it makes it easier for society to ignore the needs of the sick. If you don't really have it all that bad, then accessibility isn't actually about creating a just world but actually "special treatment"—and the need for financial support in the form of disability payments is just people being lazy.

Many people are also afraid of their empathy. They don't want to make things worse by letting people know that what is happening to them is terrible. But sometimes, that is exactly what we as patients need—someone to look us in the eye and say: "That really sucks."

What I am going through sucks. It is not pleasant. This is not true of all disability, and we have to be careful not to put our own biases regarding what people should be able to do on others and ignore their own experiences. For many people with disabilities, the impairment comes not from their lack of sight or hearing, but from our society's inability to deal with it. Many—though certainly not all—disabled people, when asked what they would wish for, would wish for the world to be easier for them to navigate than for their individual condition to be different. Be careful that sometimes when you think about how sad you would be in such a situation, you don't condescendingly put your own feelings on someone else's shoulder.

In dealing with the good intentions that turn out to be harmful and hurtful, it is the person with the illness or disability who is expected to maintain composure and to be kind and grateful to the abled person ignoring their feelings. It doesn't matter that what you are saying might actually be hurting me in some way, I am still expected to react with gratitude. My response to that is simple: I don't have the time or energy to babysit your feelings about my illness or disability, I am too busy just trying to survive either literally or figuratively.

26 Despair and Diagnosis

I went back to Ottawa, awaiting the referral to a GI. I missed the first two weeks of classes, so, on top of everything else, I was starting the semester at a disadvantage. I had notified my professors of what was going on, and many of them had kindly passed along the initial course material and assignments to me. Still, with my illness as bad as it was, I was hoping that the referral would come soon. When it finally came, I was despaired to find out that the closest appointment I could get would be in eight months. No matter who I called, the answer was always the same: our next appointment is in eight months.

I spent every day struggling between powering through extreme nausea and getting enough to eat, and then struggling more to keep even the smallest morsel down. Every day I was throwing up not just food but also yellow bile. I couldn't even brush my teeth for fear that I would have to spend the next twenty minutes bent over a toilet bowl. I continued to lose weight at an alarming rate. The flesh was melting from my bones as my body digested fat stores and muscle for fuel. In eight months, without a diagnosis and adequate treatment, I would be dead or on life support.

While I had some idea of what was wrong with me, my time spent awaiting an official diagnosis was some of the worst of my life. With every trip to the bathroom, I could feel my life force draining out of me. I was constantly exhausted. I napped more than a cat and was still always tired and chilly. No matter how hot the weather was, my skin was always cold to the touch, and I frequently shivered. My body didn't have the energy necessary to warm itself. I had to take frequent scalding baths just to feel warm.

Some days, after throwing up another meal, I would be forced to lie on the floor of the bathroom, too weak to even lift myself. I knew that I was flushing my life down the toilet and there was nothing I could do to stop it. Eating became a battle of wills, as I lay still lest a movement provoke vomiting.

Throughout it all, I dragged myself continuously to class, unwilling to fall further behind. More than once, I had to bolt out of a classroom to be sick or to use the bathroom. Taking the bus was torment as I worried that I would be sick or have an accident on my way to or from school.

The month that I arrived back in Ottawa, I had an appointment with the rheumatologist referred by the Toronto specialist to continue my follow-up care for my hip. When he saw my condition, he told me to leave the referral to him. Two days later, I got a phone call from one of the leading Crohn's and colitis doctors in Ottawa. When I say that my rheumatologist saved my life, I say so without an ounce of hyperbole.

The GI took a look at my file and told me that the tests run by the other doctor wouldn't be enough. The other doctor had not gone far enough with the colonoscopy to be diagnostically relevant, so I needed another one. In the space of one month, I would have twice a procedure that was usually reserved for older men in their 50s.

This time the procedure was done in hospital. The waiting room was actually also the recovery room. It is also where they started the IV that would give me sedation, and where I would wake up when everything was done. Sedation has the curious effect of causing mild memory loss. Even if you manage to stay awake during the procedure, chances are you won't remember much when you "sober up" so to speak. I don't remember moving from the comfortable chairs of the waiting room to the gurney. I don't remember the procedure, or coming back to the recovery room. What I will never forget however was coming to in one of those selfsame chairs, with the doctor standing in front of me. He uttered the words that I had been both dreading and waiting for.

"You have Crohn's."

He prescribed me 5-ASA, which is an oral medication similar in chemical composition to aspirin. It is one of the many treatments for Crohn's, but in my case one that we knew would be temporary. Although there is always the hope that a less intensive medication will help, with the severity of my Crohn's and preexisting autoimmune condition that required biologics, it was meant as a stopgap until he could arrange for section 8 approval for Humira.

Humira is another biologic similar to Enbrel but, unlike Enbrel, it is approved to treat both Crohn's and arthritis. When I met with my rheumatologist again, he warned me that sometimes this drug would work only on one condition but not the other, or it would provide some relief of symptoms for both conditions, but not be successful in putting both in remission.

27 A New Normal

Over the next few months, I struggled with trying to go to class while still being very sick. The medication I was given didn't help much, but I was able to develop coping techniques that made it possible for me to keep some of my food down.

On multiple occasions I had to run out of a classroom, stricken with the sudden urge to go to the bathroom. A lot of people without irritable bowel disorders assume that the disease feels like a cold or a hangover because that is all they have to compare it to. They hear digestive issues and they assume it is a mild stomach ache, occasional feeling of discomfort and nausea, followed by occasional vomiting. They might imagine a particularly bad flu, but it never seems like a big deal. What they don't realize is that, while the symptoms might be similar, the difference is that when you have the flu, you know it will eventually end. It might last a long time, but eventually, it will stop. You will get better. With Crohn's, you don't have that guarantee. You hope that eventually the meds you take will make you go into remission, but you have no guarantee. Your whole life revolves around your disease.

The feeling of needing to go to the bathroom isn't just the pressure you get when you've held it too long; rather, it is a five-second warning. You have to go to the bathroom *right now* and, if you don't, the world will end in a terrifying explosion of doom and molten lava. Add to that the fact that it can also be accompanied by severe pain and cramping, and it is an understatement to say that it is unpleasant. On some occasions, the warning might come too late. If there isn't a bathroom nearby, hopefully a change of underwear is available. Crohn's patients live in mortal fear of farting. Never before has such a simple bodily function felt more like a life or death lottery. Your body is your enemy as you do everything you can to save yourself from embarrassment.

When you have Crohn's and you feel the need to go to the washroom, you run! On one such occasion, when I felt those ominous rumbles, I got up and I ran out of the classroom, knowing that the nearest bathroom was a good three hundred meters away. What I hadn't expected was for the teacher to shoot out of the classroom after me. She called my name and caught up to me, asking me if everything was alright. I was bouncing from foot to foot, told her I had to go to the bathroom and that I would explain further after class. I made it in time, and later explained my circumstances to my professor. It was then that I realized that I was better off warning all my teachers at the beginning of every semester.

In the next few months, I learned what it feels like to be a public spectacle. The need to throw up would strike at inopportune moments, often when I was in public. I have spent at least a part of an evening out with friends locked in the bathroom, on my knees, bringing up the fries everyone else was raving about. I learned some tricks, like the fact that meat was one of the few things I would rarely bring up. I have never thrown up a well-cooked steak.

One of the worst feelings was when I needed to throw up in a public place, away from a washroom. Sometimes I was lucky and the urge would hit on the small forest path by my house that served as bus access. It was private and I was able to maintain some measure of discreetness. Other times, I was less lucky. I have had the dubious pleasure of throwing up some bright yellow udon noodles on the Department of National Defence building near the Rideau Centre. It wasn't a political statement, but rather impossible to avoid. I couldn't find a trashcan and not wanting to be sick on the areas populated by pedestrians and people waiting for the bus, I aimed for the wall.

On another occasion, I was crossing a busy street in order to get to a store. A quarter of the way across, I had to decide whether to dash back the way I came, or try to make it to the other side and risk being sick in the middle of the street. I chose safety and went back the way I came. The street corner happened to have a conveniently placed rock that I could hold onto and hide behind while I brought up my lunch. A woman in the nearby parking lot saw me and started to panic. She came over asking in a worried voice whether I needed an ambulance. She was flustered and seemed a little panicked. The last thing I wanted was a scene, but this woman was among the first people to ever show concern and I couldn't scoff at that. But how to explain to someone who is freaking out that this is a normal part of your life? That you have a disease that sometimes makes you throw up in public without any control? How do you then convince that woman that no, you don't need a hospital? "I have morning sickness," I answered.

Nausea becomes the center of your entire life. You exist only to prevent yourself from being sick. You become scared to brush your teeth. The back and forth movement of the toothbrush would provoke my gag reflex. Many mornings were spent bringing up sour bile because I tried to practice good oral hygiene. You know toilets almost intimately. You learn that the most gleaming bowl can have a harsh smell. You learn the taste of bile. Sometimes you chose your meals based on what will taste the best coming back up. Some days you schedule around meals, since you know that for a period of time after eating, you will lie as still as possible, concentrating on keeping it down. Any movement can mean the difference between nausea and outright vomiting.

Crohn's affects more than just how often you go to the bathroom and your ability to keep down food. Your entire digestive system becomes inflamed. As the colonoscopy had revealed, the entire length of my intestines was covered with bleeding ulcers. The sight of blood in the toilet became a regular occurrence. From day to day, you judge the amount of blood you are losing to determine whether it is in the normal range or whether you should be going to the hospital.

My mouth was filled with painful canker sores, which would burn every time I was sick, ate, or drank anything. Since any food I managed to keep down was still not digesting properly, I frequently developed scabs in the corner of my mouth from vitamin deficiencies. Those scabs would crack and bleed whenever I opened my mouth.

Some weeks were better than others. During some weeks, I could almost believe that I had the situation under control, and that things were getting better and I could go back to normal. I could do things like go to class, or do my homework. Good days were those when brushing my teeth didn't make me throw up bile.

28 Hollow

Near the end of the semester, my symptoms took a turn for the worse. Almost every meal ended up down the drain. I knew I had to do something soon. I had an assignment I had been looking forward to in my Victorian literature class; I was to do a seminar comparing Frankenstein and his monster to the mythical figure of Prometheus. I really wanted the chance to present. Despite having not kept food down in close to two weeks, I decided to give the seminar and immediately afterward headed to the ER. The thrill of presenting helped me ignore my symptoms for the brief half hour I was up there.

Once class was over, I handed in my essay and started out the door. My professor, one of my favorites, wanted to congratulate me on the great job I had done. Imagine her surprise when I confided that I had to go to the hospital.

At the ER, the triage nurse asked me why I was there. I answered that I needed to be admitted, put on IV fluids, and given prednisone until the flare calmed down. The nurse gave me a sideways look and made some comment about waiting to see what the doctor had to say. The doctor, it seemed, agreed with me. In a matter of hours, I was put on IV and brought upstairs. They started me on an IV form of medication. I was in hospital for close to a week before I was able to keep food down. I was also given prednisone again, this time in a much higher dose than I had had previously.

In the hospital, stuffed full of painkillers, antinausea agents, and other drugs, I didn't notice the peculiar effects of prednisone. Prednisone is a steroid that is often prescribed for autoimmune patients on a temporary basis. It works aggressively; I saw that firsthand back in St. Catharines when the swelling in my ankles went down.

In the long term, the steroid has severe side effects that make it unsuited to continued use. The one that concerned me most was the degradation of hip joints. When I got home from the hospital, away from the soporific effects of those other drugs, I was filled with an unnatural sick sort of energy. My whole body felt strung tight, like an overtuned guitar string; I was vibrating, but felt like at any moment I would snap. At times I had to lie down for fear of falling over. My whole face would be flushed from it all. This translated into difficulty sleeping. At one point I cleaned the whole bathroom from top to bottom, made cookies and muffins, and did the dishes, all at two in the morning.

Sometimes the sick energy only infects one part of your body, like your legs. Your mind, arms, stomach, back could all be aching tired, but your legs would be unable to stay still. You would lay down at three in the morning, desperate to sleep, but your legs would be ice cold and unable to stop moving. The covers would bounce from your inability to keep your toe from tapping. Since your legs need to keep moving you cannot find a comfortable position to lie in, or even sit in. Of course, three in the morning is not a time that a young woman can safely walk around outside. You can forget about taking the overeager dog for a walk or getting something productive done. Wandering the apartment corridors is too inconsiderate to the neighbors. You find yourself instead wearing a groove in the carpet as you take advantage of the semiopen layout of your apartment: dining room, living room, hallway, and kitchen, over and over and over again, reversing direction from time to time in some faint desire to eliminate the dizziness that you pretend is the result of the circles. All in the desperate hope that you can tire out your legs, or perhaps at least get the blood moving down into them to warm them up. The skin of your legs is ice cold, because despite the rapid heart rate and high blood pressure, your circulation is no good. Hot baths, heating packs, layers of clothing, nothing helps. You continue to feel cold no matter what.

Another symptom is that such a situation makes you gain weight. For those of you familiar with starvation in any way, you might know that, when the body is denied food for a long period of time, one of its first reactions is to store as much fat as it can. Add to that a steroid whose purpose in part is to promote weight gain, and you end up with a deadly spiral into obesity. You do your best to avoid the temptation to overeat, but the false hunger gnaws at you. You are never comfortable. When you are eating, you feel like the pressure on the side of your stomach as though you have eaten too much, and yet when you stop the void beckons. The fact that you have not been able to eat comfortably for the last several months only makes things worse. When every bite you eat has to be so carefully monitored and considered, the sudden freedom to indulge can be overwhelming. If you do manage to fill the void, it is too much. The prednisone masks your satiety so that by the time you have noticed, you're too full. You find yourself with the back of your throat burning, as your body debates the merits of throwing up.

The drug leaves me with the sensation of being always full and somehow always starving. I compare it to the feeling of having a balloon, which I always imagine as being red, blown to large proportions in my stomach. It presses against the sides and expands the organ, but still, the stomach is essentially hollow and begging to be filled.

Along with the prednisone, I was sent a referral for starting Humira. In early December, I met with the nurse who would show me how to use the new auto-injector. By some strange coincidence, the pharmacy ran out of the auto-injector the day I picked up my prescription, and I was left with the syringes. The nurse, knowing I had used Enbrel before, took care of the first round of shots. The helpful benefits of Humira did not come as fast as Enbrel, especially while I was taking prednisone. Still, I did observe some positive effect. I hoped I was out of the woods and could focus fully on my schooling once more.

29 Learning How to Eat

Over the next several months, I began to relearn how to eat and what to eat. Crohn's is unique in that trigger foods vary from person to person. I had a classmate with Crohn's who could not eat tomatoes or any acidic foods. For me, acidity wasn't a problem. Instead, foods that triggered gas production caused the most pain. No longer could I happily sip cider on cold fall evenings, not unless I wanted to be curled up in pain a few hours later. Sweet potatoes, beans, and other such foods could only be eaten on rare occasions, and only in small amounts. I also had to say goodbye to milk and yogurt.

Although I had always had mild anemia, low iron content in my blood, the bleeding caused by ulcerations in my intestines made it much worse. In weeks when I didn't have red meat, I would have painful cramps that would make my leg constrict. When I chanced to see the pictures from my colonoscopy, the inside of my intestines looked like someone had taken a cheese grater to them. They were striped with lines of blood.

Eating was a lot like playing a lottery. Just because a food may have been okay to eat the day before, didn't mean that it would be okay the next. Sometimes, even the way in which food was prepared could change its effect on you. Texture, consistency, smell, seasoning, taste can all change whether eating something is safe or not. There are moments when even the foods that never set you off can still be too much. It becomes a battle just to eat something, since your first instinct is to stay away from anything that you can either eat or smell. Favorite foods that just a moment before tasted and smelled so appetizing will suddenly stick in your throat and have you wondering whether you need to run to the washroom.

Smell can be a trigger, too. Everyday tasks like taking out the garbage, picking up after pets, doing groceries, or walking down the street can become a risk. Sometimes an odor can mean the difference between being fine and being crouched down on the ground spilling out your guts. On those days, you want to avoid going anywhere lest your overly sensitive stomach strike at an inopportune moment.

Along the same vein, I have often experienced very strange cravings related to my Crohn's symptoms. When my nausea was at its peak, I would dream of sour candy. Something about the sourness soothed me and made me feel a little less sick. But there was a balance that needed to be maintained, because too much would burn my mouth. Sometimes a craving presents itself as an overwhelming taste in the back of my mouth, one that won't go away until I hit just the right taste note. Experience lets me know what taste corresponds to what food, but how do I explain that urgency to someone else?

30 Immunosuppressed

While the Humira seemed to be working for the first few months, it wasn't long before I started getting flare symptoms in the days preceding my next injection. I gave myself the shot once every two weeks, and the few days before the next injection came with increased bathroom trips and nausea, if not outright vomiting.

Worse yet, the injections impaired my immune system to a larger extent than the previous drugs. I caught colds more often than ever before. Whenever I was sick, I would have to wait until I got better before giving myself the next shot. Imagine existing in this continuous cycle of colds and digestive problems. Even relatively healthy weeks were draining.

The following fall was the year of the swine flu scare. Everywhere you went you would see people wearing masks, and big signs telling people to wash their hands to prevent the spread of H1N1. The University of Ottawa suffered its own outbreak, which culminated with the death of a chemistry teacher. With the high fatality rate of the disease and my lowered immune system, I was worried about exposure. When I started feeling flu-like symptoms, I thought it best to go to the doctor and get myself checked out.

One strange aspect of my health that was only encouraged by the immunosuppressants was my tendency not to get fevers, even when I was sick. This backfired for me when I went to the doctor since he refused to admit that I was sick. Despite my insistence that this felt different from Crohn's, he was convinced that is was just a flare-up. I continued going to class. When after another week I still felt sick, I went back. Still no fever meant that I still could not be sick. The week afterward I got a bit of a break. I felt better enough to give myself my shot. Within days, I was sick again.

This time, I didn't bother with the clinic. I went to the hospital and they confirmed what I had already suspected. I had swine flu. In the end, I missed close to two months of class as I struggled to get over it. I also suffered from the guilt of having gone to class while I was sick. I was convinced that I had contributed to the spread of the illness at the university.

Having the flu and having a Crohn's flare at the same time was torturous. Those two months seem like a haze. I spent countless hours zonked out. One morning, I woke up with the feeling that I was drowning. I couldn't breathe, my lungs filled with liquid. I coughed as hard as I could, trying to bring up whatever was blocking my airways. I ran to the washroom and vomited up a glop of phlegm. The gasp that followed the expulsion of that stuff almost burned, but the air had never tasted sweeter. At the hospital, the staff expressed their shock over the fact that I had managed to get rid of the fluid in my lungs. For many people, that feeling of drowning was the last thing they felt.

31 Let's Talk about Vaccines

I want to take this moment to mention vaccinations. In this specific case, I got sick before the vaccine for swine flu was widely available. After I recovered, my parents mentioned that our doctor back in St. Catharines was walking around with the shot in his pocket, so that if he saw me he could give it to me right away. He was concerned for me and the possibility of me getting sick again. While I am pretty sure the doctor was joking, especially with the risk of the vaccine spoiling no matter how cold the weather, eventually I got the shot. One of few that I am able to take.

Immunosuppressants limit your ability to get vaccinated. There is a whole list of shots that are considered "live-vaccines" that you cannot take. Even when you are vaccinated, you are still at risk. Vaccines work by enhancing your body's immunity against a disease. If you are like most people, this means you will never get sick from that disease—or, if you do, it will be significantly less severe with a smaller chance of complications. For those of us with compromised immune systems, even an enhanced immunity might not be enough as our bodies simply cannot fight off the illness. We depend on herd (or community) immunity.

For us, the antivaccination movement is particularly scary. Every child who doesn't get their shots, every adult who neglects to get their boosters, contributes to a trend that may one day kill me. Whenever the news tells of a new outbreak of some previously disappearing disease like measles or whooping cough, I wonder if this is the one that will lay me low.

Herd immunity depends on every person who is able getting vaccinated. With each healthy person who doesn't immunize, the barrier that protects those of us who are particularly susceptible to disease weakens and our lives are endangered. There is no excuse for diseases such as polio, whooping cough, or measles to still exist. It is within our power as a community to make them disappear and we as a society owe it to future generations to do just that. The longer these diseases are allowed to exist, the scarier they become. We are giving them the ability to evolve, to become more dangerous, and we are doing this for no other reason than because we are letting con artists and fraudsters convince us rather than listening to science and medical experts. When an actress with no medical background and who makes millions from telling her story is given more credibility on matters of health than the many doctors and scientists who actually research these areas, then we know our world is in trouble.

Becoming infected, as someone who relies on immunosuppressants to manage other conditions, carries more consequences than just coming down with something. Swine flu, although not the least of my worries, was not the only one. In order to fight off the infection, I had to delay the next dose. The delays in medicating myself for my Crohn's also had an adverse effect on my hip. I began to limp more frequently and the twinges in my back increased as well. The progress I had made with the joint was reversed, and my mobility became even more compromised. Added to the delays caused by health, my pharmacy had difficulties filling my prescription on time. Frequently, I would be delayed by a few days to a week before the pharmacy managed to get the next set of injections. Since the injections cost in the thousands, it was impossible for me to have a stockpile going. While I would go in a week or so in advance to order the next dose, they often still failed to have it on time.

32 New Meds

The Humira was not working. I spoke to my doctor, and we started the process of switching me to Remicade. Unlike the medication I had been taking up until then, Remicade was not an injection but rather an infusion. In the long term, the plan was to go every eight weeks at the standard dose. The introduction, however, starts with three infusions given closer together and then eventually going up to the standard frequency. Normally, there has to be a three-month separation between stopping one medication and starting another. However, due to the severity of symptoms after I completely stopped Humira, the doctor worked on getting me in for a dose as soon as possible.

The drug is given via IV in a special clinic. These clinics exist because if the drug was being administered in a hospital, the expectation would be that the hospital, or rather Ontario Health Insurance Plan (OHIP), would pay for it. Since Remicade is upward of $1,000 per 100 milligrams and the standard dose for Crohn's is 400 mg, the hospital and the province had no interest in footing the bill. The Remicade infusion clinics, however, were nicely stocked. Since an infusion can take approximately three hours, the chairs are recliners. Most people fall asleep during the infusion; the rest either read or watch TV. While the clinic is run mostly by nurses, they are usually attached to walk-in clinics or doctors' offices in the event of emergency. Some people experience allergic reactions like hives, while a small minority may go into full anaphylactic shock. For this reason, you are expected to spend an extra hour at the clinic after the first infusion for monitoring.

You learn a lot about IVs when you get them that frequently. Many patients learn about their own veins and may have a regular "Remicade vein" that they use. You learn to make sure that you drink a lot before your infusion since dehydration makes them shrink. Those of us living in colder climates learn how temperature can affect veins, and know to ask for a heating pad on cold days. Those of us who bring our computers along learn to work with an IV in our hand. You learn that keeping your arm and wrist straight can make a huge difference in how long your infusion takes. Some of us learn the difference between a needle piercing skin, muscle, nerve, or vein. And for many of us, we learn to look forward to getting our IVs since it can mean relief.

The Remicade worked. It worked fast. Within weeks, I already felt much better. In the years following my first infusion, my symptoms have mostly calmed down. This is not to say that I am healed, but rather that I no longer feel like I am dying every day.

I still have to be admitted to the hospital fairly frequently, averaging about twice per year. The symptoms that admit me can vary. During one admission, my trips to the bathroom were causing me an incredible amount of pain. To put it colorfully, I felt as though someone had inserted a hot, rusty, knitting needle up my bum. Sitting was excruciating, but walking was worse. The pain, accompanied by nausea and diarrhea, finally became unbearable and I was forced to go to the emergency room.

On other occasions, I went in because I was passing too much blood and worried whether the ulcers in my colon were getting worse, or perhaps something had perforated. One time the pain in my abdomen was strong enough to cause concerns regarding my appendix or the possibility of a blockage.

While the specific symptoms that bring me to the hospital might vary, the usual treatments stay the same. I am told not to eat, put on prednisone, then gradually reintroduced to food again, usually a low residue diet: potatoes, pasta, meat loaf, and no raw vegetables.

33 Potty Training

As a Crohn's patient, you learn to live with an unpredictable bathroom schedule. As I mentioned previously, this is more than the usual urgency that comes with having to go to the washroom. It is difficult to predict when an urge will go from urgent to unstoppable, and how much time you have in between. On many forums where people discuss how to deal with the illness, it is recommended to always travel with a change of underwear. While this is good advice, the reality is that in order to truly be safe you would have to travel with a change of underwear, pants, socks, wet wipes, a plastic bag, and toilet paper. If you have the space, you should also pack a port-a-potty. Since carrying all of that everywhere you go isn't exactly practical, the most useful thing you can pack is a sense of humor and a strong stomach for embarrassment.

My first bathroom accident happened on campus, in the middle of a midterm. This semester in particular had been somewhat difficult for me. The building in which a good chunk of my classes were located was under construction and had only one working washroom. Still, as luck would have it, this washroom happened to be on my classroom's floor. For most of the semester, everything was mostly okay, but on the day of the midterm, I woke up feeling a little ill. I sat down for the exam and began writing. At some point, I could feel the urge hitting me and received permission to go to the washroom. I made my usual dash, only to discover that the construction crew had finally made it to my classroom's floor. Both the women's and men's room were closed for construction. In a panic, I tried to determine the nearest washroom and realized it was in the bottom level of the adjacent building. When I got to the other building, I had to decide whether the wait for the elevator outweighed the risk of walking down stairs. I ran down the stairs, hoping I could hold it in. I couldn't risk the possibility of being crowded into a tiny box while my ability to stay clean was so much in question.

This time, I was not lucky. Imagine, if you will, the overwhelming embarrassment of being an adult and having an accident like that in public. Even if you're lucky, like I was, that nothing made it to the floor, imagine the horror as you wonder if everyone around you can smell it.

I finally made it to a stall and used toilet paper to clean myself up as best I could. I scrubbed helplessly at my underwear in the sink, hoping that no one would walk in to see what I was doing. I was in such shock that I couldn't even cry. Once I had cleaned myself up enough to leave the bathroom, I trudged back upstairs to tell my professor that I would be unable to finish the midterm. He had figured out something was wrong when I was gone as long as I was. I feel really lucky that he expressed understanding. I don't know what I would have done if he had threatened me with failure for not finishing the exam.

I walked in shock back to my girlfriend's apartment, where I was staying during the week. I considered the possibility of going back to my own apartment, fearing that, if she saw me, she wouldn't find me sexy anymore. I didn't want to see the disgust in her eyes, wondering to myself if our every future interaction would be tainted with the unsubtle odor of "unclean." This was my reality. This was something that could happen again. Would she be able to handle that?

I knew that taking a half hour bus back to my apartment was out of the question, and so I had to risk staying. I am lucky that Alex is a wonderful woman. Far outside my fear of rejection, Alex took me in her arms and wrapped me in her robe. While I showered, she washed my clothes for me and readied some food and a funny movie to cheer me up. She spent the rest of the evening cuddling me and helping me to forget about what had happened.

The fear of rejection is something many people with chronic illness and disabilities struggle with. There is this idea in our culture that having a chronic illness is a personal failing of some kind, whether that illness is something to do with mental health or physical health. It ties in with the "just world" fallacy—that bad things must be deserved in some way. This is why, whenever someone is sick, there is this belief that they must have done *something* wrong. Otherwise, life is just a lottery. People fear what they cannot control, and so much of health is out of our hands. Even though we might know what causes certain illnesses, we don't always know how to prevent them. What makes one person who has the gene that leads to Crohn's get sick, while someone else with the same gene doesn't? If two people live the same life, with the same habits, the same diet, what makes one of them get cancer and the other not?

This is why the alternative medicine business is so lucrative despite the lack of evidence that it works. Like religion, it sells the illusion of control. In a world of fear and uncertainty, the illusion of control can be as reassuring as actually having it. When the illusion is the only thing available, it makes it doubly hard to resist.

34 *Living* with an Invisible Disability

When you are going through the process of discovery and diagnosis, your life reads like a narrative as you drift from one discovery or major event to the next. There is always this hope of that happy ending. At some point, however, chronic illness and disability become your life, and you realize that there will be no ending at all. Rather, the story of your illness just becomes the story of you. Major events still stand out, but they are almost lost among the daily minutiae of having a chronic illness. More importantly, narrative implies change.

One of the harshest and most painful realities of living every day with a chronic illness or invisible disability is that very little changes from day to day. It is true that in the long run things might get better or worse, and that the level of symptoms from day to day might change, but the debilitation is constant.

One thing that a lot of people don't understand about such conditions is that, for many, pain is a constant companion. Days completely without pain are either exceedingly rare, or simply don't exist. Most days, your pain remains at a fairly consistent level. Like the hum from a fluorescent light, you notice it from time to time, but you learn to ignore it after a while. These are the days when you manage to get things done, although it drains your energy just the same. Sometimes something brings your attention to it, and so you become aware of the pain again. Sometimes, other things make you more sensitive to it: a stressful day, not feeling well, different types of pain like a headache or cramps, etc. These triggers can suddenly make you more aware of your pain, make it more difficult to ignore. Like the humming of the light, it didn't get any louder but you are more sensitive to it in those times.

Unlike the lights, however, the pain can get louder or more severe. Some days the pain isn't just more noticeable, it is actually more intense. The pain can spread to other parts of your body. In the case of my arthritis, the pain might spread from my damaged hip to the other one, and it might spread to my knees, or spine, or ribs, or any other joint in my body. It can change in how it is perceived by shifting from a dull ache to a sharp pinching or throbbing sensation.

Any of these changes are felt more acutely because they differ from the norm. In the case of Crohn's it can mean that the pain has affected a different part of my digestive system. It can mean that rather than my usual ache around my stomach area and mid abdomen, I suddenly feel a sharp pain in my left side. Or perhaps I might get intense cramps in my lower belly or spasms in my intestines. Any shift or change in pain can suddenly bring the whole weight of it crashing down on your body.

Sometimes the pain is not necessarily recognizable as pain. For example, some mornings when my Crohn's hits me particularly hard, I get the sensation of being able to actually feel my intestines. It doesn't matter whether the bowel movement is loose or solid. Explaining how something like this feels can be extremely difficult since the majority of people have nothing to compare it to. In some ways, I suppose, it is similar to the feeling you get when you urgently have to go to the bathroom. Added to that is a feeling of irritation, like skin that has been rubbed raw or a diaper rash, except all of this feeling is in a part of the body that people are not usually consciously aware of. There's also a burning sensation, similar to what many people experience when eating very spicy food.

When this happens, I can feel the movements of my intestines, and the bowel movement sticking to the walls of my gut. There is a feeling like lemon juice on an exposed wound. It feels like I have to go to the bathroom, but an actual trip will often yield only mucus. Yet I keep going, because experience has taught me that "nature's call" is never safe to ignore.

The feeling can last for as little as an hour, or as long as the entire morning, sometimes even longer. It makes concentration nearly impossible. Sitting is uncomfortable, especially since using toilet paper during each of the frequent bathroom trips results in rawness. Overall the experience may not conform to what is classically considered pain, but the result and the discomfort is the same. There is also always a risk that this feeling will turn into more acute pain down the line.

Whether I am having a bad pain day or a normal pain day, one constant is the effect it has on my energy level. The effort, subconscious or otherwise, involved in ignoring or managing pain is a continual drain on resources. Every task, regardless of how small, has to be taken into account in a mental calculation of my daily allotment of energy. Even enjoyable tasks have to be factored into that equation. Consider a bath, for example: the heat can provide some much needed relief from pain and be relaxing. In order to take one, however, you have to get up, pour the water, get undressed, make sure you have a towel, and so on. These may seem like simple or basic tasks, bet they require an output of energy that may simply not be available. The rewards of an action must always be balanced against their costs.

To complicate matters further, the energy reserves that I have to draw on change from day to day, making my reward/cost equation inconsistent and unpredictable. Just because I might have been able to go to work, come home, make dinner, and get some cleaning done yesterday, does not guarantee that I will be able to do all that today, or even tomorrow. Similarly, the energy required to complete a task can also change. Whereas one day, boiling a pot of water for noodles can be a relatively low-energy activity, on other days, the task can seem beyond my reach. Different factors impact what the level of energy output required will be. On days when my overall energy level is already dangerously low, every activity feels as though it requires twice as much energy to complete.

Imagine energy as a glass of water and each activity as a sip. When you have a full glass, although each sip lowers the overall level of water, the impact is less noticeable than when you start with only half a glass. When your glass is only half full, each one of those sips takes a greater percentage of the overall total. How quickly you run out of water also changes, so you have to ration your sips more carefully and over a greater period of time. You are forced to work with less and so how much you get is also less.

Your energy level for the day can also be hidden from you. You don't realize how much you started with until you have almost nothing left. You start your day thinking it will be a high-energy day and plan accordingly. You take a little extra effort getting ready for work, you plan to make a more elaborate meal, you take on an extra task during the day, or you promise to have something done earlier than expected. Then midday comes and you realize that you overestimated your level of strength or energy for the day. You have to reevaluate how much you are capable of. This might mean missing a deadline, or having to cancel on a friend. It can mean putting the defrosting meat back in the fridge for a few days, or asking your partner to take over one of your chores for the day. Every little failing like that cuts at your self-confidence, making you doubt yourself and your abilities. During your next high-energy day, you might take on less thinking you won't be able to finish. Or alternately, you take on even more, feeling guilty and needing to make up for your inabilities.

If you take on too much, you could be paying back that energy debt over the next several days. Energy debts can be paid back as illness, pain, flare-ups, or exhaustion. There are no set rules as to how long you will be paying back the debt. Energy debts and pain debts come with high interest; you can be paying back one moment of poor judgment for days, weeks, or even months.

This inability to judge your ability to handle tasks from day to day can make it very difficult to work and maintain a livable salary. It is no coincidence that people coping with disabilities often struggle with unemployment and poverty.

Part 3: Disability and Social Justice

35 Identifying as Disabled

It might seem strange, but I went a long time without identifying as disabled.

When I first started getting sick, my end goal was to get better. It was to get back to what life used to be like before I got sick. I always looked at everything that was wrong with me and kept thinking, "Someday I won't be like this. Someday I will be normal." I spent the next few years after that working on achieving just that. I don't know at what point I realized that I would never "get better." It didn't necessarily come as some giant revelation. At some point I just realized that I was no longer going into things hoping "this will cure me" but instead was thinking "this will make my symptoms less severe."

Even after I realized that there was no "getting better" for me, I still resisted the impulse to consider myself "disabled." I don't know how often I would catch myself saying things along the lines of, "Oh, I have a disability, yes, but you know I'm not *disabled*." There was more to it than just wanting to believe that I could get better someday. I was afraid that people would judge me, but beyond that I also felt like people wouldn't believe me.

There are two sides to the label "disabled."

We as a society have a very specific concept of what disability means. Anyone with a disability who falls outside this concept must be faking it. If you need a wheelchair, for example, you better always be using it, because you shouldn't be able to walk at all. You are not allowed to use a wheelchair if you only can't walk sometimes, or it if hurts to walk, or if sometimes you can manage with a cane. If you are blind and use a white cane, you better be completely blind. Our society has this concept of disability as being all or nothing.

It creates a binary: "disabled" and "not disabled," with one side being heavily defined. In turn, anyone who doesn't conform 100 percent to that definition must be fake taking advantage of the system. The problem of course with such an assertion, as with any binary really, is that it is not a complete or even accurate picture of the world.

Many people with disabilities have fluctuating symptoms. In my case, for example, most days I can walk unaided. I might limp from time to time, but otherwise I am okay. However, on other days I might require the use of a cane. On other days, the pain might get bad enough that I require the use of a wheelchair to get around. This doesn't make my disability "not real," nor does it mean I am faking it when I am in a wheelchair. Many of my other impairments are also not visible to most people. When I go to the washroom three times in the space of an hour, that is me living with my disability as much as when I am throwing up in public or when I don't make it to the washroom in time. When my abdominal pain makes it impossible for me to concentrate, that is also a manifestation of my disability.

What this binary does is make it more difficult for people who need services to access them, while making it easier for those in power to ignore us. If the only people who count as being disabled are those with easy-to-identify symptoms, then those in power can pretend that accessibility is not as big an issue or requirement as it is. (Though frankly even if the only people who were disabled were those with obvious and identifiable disabilities, accessibility would still be an important consideration.)

In effect, on the one side, you have people with legitimate disabilities feeling like they are not entitled to consider themselves disabled. On the other side, meanwhile, factors conspire to create fear about identifying as disabled.

We as a society have this concept that people with disabilities, especially those receiving disability assistance, are lazy, sad, and pathetic. That they are deserving of pity. There is an underlying current of society that holds the belief that the words "I am disabled" actually mean "my life is not worth living." In a culture that prioritizes what any given person can do and how productive they are, it is not surprising that this is the case. Our worth is dictated by how useful we are, and people with disabilities are assumed to be useless to society as a whole.

There is active pressure from society on those with disabilities to not identify as disabled; this pressure comes with the message that "being disabled" is a bad thing. It is this same impulse that leads friends and family to say such patronizing things as, "The only disability is a bad attitude" or "You're not sick, you just need to think positive." They cannot understand why we would do something so "negative" like be disabled or, worse yet, talk about being disabled. For me, finally admitting to myself and eventually the world that "yes, I am disabled" was incredibly liberating.

36 What It Really Means to Be Poor and Disabled

It took less than thirty minutes for Ontario Works to decide that I don't qualify for welfare. (Well, it took them an hour and a half if you count the hour I was on hold.) Thirty minutes to decide that even though the money my noncitizen wife makes is not enough to cover all of our bills, it is too much for us to qualify for financial assistance. Our bills are not outrageous, but the reality these days is that life is expensive. Housing, transportation, communication, food—it all adds up. All the while prices continue to increase as the income I can reasonably expect to make decreases.

Half an hour is better, I suppose, than the six months that the Ontario Disability Support Payments (ODSP), what in the United States would be called disability, took to say no. According to them, having extreme pain, not being able to walk long distances or stand for long periods of time, regularly bleeding internally, and not being able to keep food down or stay out of the bathroom for more than an hour, all while coming down with frequent viral and bacterial infections due to being immunosuppressed, doesn't count as a disability. Of course not! Why would something that puts you in the hospital and causes you to be hooked up to IV nutrients, steroids, and painkillers every few months or weeks count as a disability? It is not like being in pain, or in the hospital, or not having the energy to move because you haven't digested food in days, impacts your ability to work. Of course *not*!

Those who are sick or have disabilities are particularly vulnerable to becoming trapped by poverty. When the measure of personal worth is closely tied to productivity, those who may struggle to hold a job—or even just to get out of bed in the mornings—because of chronic illness or disability are made to feel useless, worthless. If you are poor with frequent medical needs and expenses, society tells you every day that you may not be worth keeping alive.

For me, it all started with my disabilities. Before that, I was a typical broke student. I wasn't rich by any means, but my poverty was expected, and temporary. My parents paid my bills, and they gave me a weekly allowance for groceries. Budgeting meant deciding how much of that weekly allowance went for treats and how much for essentials. It meant making sure that my monthly bills didn't go over a certain agreed-upon amount per month. It meant looking for a job to supplement that support and help take some of the burden off of my parents. But, ultimately, it meant that if I ever got in trouble, if I ever had an unexpected expense or if something bad happened, I had a safety net to fall back on. I had parents who would make sure I wouldn't starve or go homeless. Who, while letting me learn from my mistakes (like making me pay off my maxed-out credit card myself), would also not let me become desperate.

When my health troubles started, so did more serious concerns about money. For example, the biologic I was put on may have helped modulate my immune system in order to help prevent the immune response that was causing the problems in the first place, but, as a new type of drug, it was also extremely expensive. At first, the cost was a hardship but manageable, and my parents were able to cover the expense.

For months, my parents and I tried to get on Trillium, a provincial prescription insurance that takes an applicant's financial information into consideration. While we were approved, they decided to take my parent's income into consideration and the deductible was so high that the coverage was essentially nonexistent. This is a common occurrence. Despite the fact that my parents lived more than eight hours away, it made no difference in Trillium's considerations.

When my Crohn's kicked in, I was switched from biologic to biologic, finally ending up on Remicade. Had it ended there, my family might have been able to continue supporting me. This was not the case, however. My Crohn's refused to go into remission. I was getting better, but that only meant that I was no longer ending up in the hospital every two weeks. Rather, I ended up being admitted into the hospital twice a year. Still, I remained sick. I was able to simply survive my flares until the next dose, experiencing brief windows of seeming normality immediately after my infusions. As a result, my doctor decided that something more extreme had to be done to try and push my system into remission. I would have to go on a double dose of Remicade.

For those who don't know, Remicade is given as an IV usually every eight weeks. A standard dose for Crohn's is 400 mg with weight being taken into consideration. This dose costs approximately $4,000. *Four Thousand Dollars.* My doctor increased my dose to 1,000 mg every six weeks. That is $10,000 every six weeks. Who among you could comfortably spend that much money every two months? Not my parents and certainly not me. The only way I could afford that medication would be if I got Trillium coverage. The only way to manage that was to stop being my parents' dependant. That is to say, in order to get medication that was, without exaggeration, keeping me alive, I would have to give up the financial security of accepting help from my parents.

My first double dose would be given before I could qualify for Trillium. With that in mind, I did something I had been hoping to avoid for a long period of time: I took out a student loan. More accurately, I took out a student line of credit. I used the money from the line of credit to pay for my double dose. I also used it to help pay expenses until I could find a job that would cover my living expenses. I was officially on my own.

37 Becoming Poor

I found a job in a real estate office that would help cover my expenses. I was prepared to work hard. I wanted to keep this job until I was finished with school and could start my long-term career. I knew it would be difficult, but I was prepared to apply myself and be the perfect employee. At this point, I still saw myself on the path to middle-class normalcy: a little difficulty in the beginning followed by relative comfort and security in a white-collar job. I didn't want to be a millionaire or a CEO, just to own a home, have a family, have a job I could like well enough, be able to go on the occasional vacation, put a little money away for retirement . . . I was prepared to have to save for a few months when I wanted to make some little luxury purchase, but my life, my home, my security would not be at risk. I still dream of all those things.

What I didn't know was that my new job would send me on a path that would eventually make my illness quite a bit worse.

It started out great. It was work I enjoyed, and there was a lot of variety; I might be asked to come up with an event idea, file papers with the court, plan a meal, do social media marketing, write, do clerical work, etc. I was having fun and feeling stimulated.

A few months into my job, however, trouble started brewing. My boss was considering a company move, and her assistant had to devote herself to the paperwork side of the business. She looked for someone new, but eventually, the responsibilities the assistant no longer had time for simply fell to me. I didn't mind since more work meant more hours and, in turn, more pay. Soon, however, it was clear that the amount of work expected was beyond what was feasible. I was doing the work of a marketing assistant, a clerical assistant, and a personal assistant, all at the same time. I often found myself working for ten to twelve hours straight. I was frequently working through lunch, or missing it all together. I would come home exhausted, too tired to do anything other than go straight to sleep.

While I was doing the work of three people, my boss believed that my work load didn't equal any more than that of half a person. She became dissatisfied with my performance, convinced that I was too slow, or just too lazy. The stress of trying to maintain the long hours and quality of performance, all while increasing the speed at which I completed everything, began to make itself felt.

I bought a car because my commute by bus was more than an hour long, and because I never knew if I would have access to the company car on any given day. With the money I was making at the time, the purchase was within our means. It gave me more opportunities to be even more helpful at work by making it possible for me to deliver things across town, but it also made me more productive at home by saving time and money on tasks such as grocery shopping and taking pets to the vet.

I was constantly anxious. I would receive multiple texts a day, from the office, from my boss, from clients. At times I would be messaged late at night to perform some emergency task. My inbox was constantly flooded. I was falling behind in my work, which in turn made my employer punish me for unproductivity. I was becoming sick more frequently, finding blood in my stool at an alarming rate. I was admitted for some time with pancreatitis. I needed my medication more and more frequently. I was constantly exhausted and felt wrung out and on the verge of a meltdown. I started gaining weight due to the stress and the unhealthy eating habits that came from rarely having enough energy to cook.

Soon after I bought my car, my boss started hinting that I might not receive my next paycheck. This made me feel so stressed that I had to take a sick day. I felt as though I couldn't breathe. I looked back over what had been happening in the last few months and realized that I was in an abusive relationship with my boss. I was having a panic attack every time I heard my phone ring. I would even jump whenever I heard someone else's phone, wondering what I had done wrong now. I felt like I was about to snap.

Finally, I realized that I could not continue living the way that I had been, and I quit. Despite all the hardships that came from that decision, I still maintain that it was the right thing to do.

I began to look for a new job right away and, eventually, I had an offer. It was a bit different from what I had done in the past. This time, I would be working as an office assistant in the trades industry. My health started deteriorating again almost immediately. The office was frequently dirty, with dust lining every surface. My bosses were constantly at each other's throats. It was not uncommon for someone to slam doors, yell, or burst into tears. The whole office environment fed on drama, with everyone talking about everyone. It was a minefield of emotional stress.

My Crohn's rebelled. Over the next several months I existed in constant pain well beyond what I had learned to tolerate. I was frequently ill. Mornings would involve me struggling to find the energy to get up and get to work. I had to call in sick frequently since the dirty environment did not agree with my immunosuppressed status. Because of my frequent illnesses, I did not receive a promised raise.

I started going to the washroom more frequently. This was remarked upon by my employers, who wondered whether such frequent trips were necessary. Though I was working significantly fewer hours than I had previously, my exhaustion worsened. After the previous work environment had set off my anxiety, this new emotionally volatile environment became too much to bear. After months of hoping everything would settle down, after weeks of looking for a new job on the side, I was admitted to the hospital with sharp, stabbing pains in my stomach.

The doctor in the emergency room remarked that my Crohn's was flaring and told me that I needed to take time off. She wrote me a doctor's note saying that I needed to stay away from work for the next week. My regular GI followed up with his own concerns about the state of my health over the last few months. It was becoming obvious that I could not keep working much longer without serious long-term consequences to my health. I needed to stop.

38 My Welfare State

I applied for temporary employment insurance government sickness benefits and left my job. I needed to rest if I wanted to have any hope of restabilizing.

Applying for sickness benefits is a difficult process on its own. It takes weeks to get approval and, in the meantime, you exist in a state of moneyless limbo. It is a terrifying situation. You are not working and have no money coming in, and you have to wait weeks to find out if you are even approved. You worry that, in the end, they will decide not to cover you and that you will be without the funds you need to pay rent, pay your bills, or buy groceries. You have no way of knowing which way the decision will go. Many people who deserve to be on sick leave don't get it, while others are approved. There's really no way to tell what your fate will be.

I spent Christmas in this state of limbo, relying on the kindness of friends who donated to the blog I had started writing a year or so before. It had started out as a place for me to post things related to my fantasy writing, like world maps and character designs. Soon, however, it became my personal blog where I wrote on issues that I found important. I responded to news articles, discussed issues related to social justice, and talked about my personal life and struggles. It is here that I first started sharing my story of what it meant to be young and sick. It was here that I made myself and my conditions less invisible. My parents sent me some money for Christmas as well, which helped to ensure that I could afford to eat, and Alex's parents also sent us some extra cash along with her tuition.

Finally, I got my approval. For the next few months, I could relax a little about money and focus on getting back to form. Still, in the back of my mind was another fear: What would I do once the temporary coverage period ran out? How long would it take me to find a new job, and would I even be able to work again? It was at this time that I applied for ODSP, permanent disability support. With disability, I wouldn't have to worry if I continued to be unable to work. All around me, people were warning me that getting approved for disability is close to impossible. As a contingency, I did my best to look for alternative sources of income that would work with my disabilities. I found another job, but my anxieties and disabilities impaired my ability to function and I was soon fired.

As noted earlier, my application for disability was initially denied after a six-month wait. Nearly a year and a half later, however, after having scheduled a court date, I was finally approved. A year and a half of living without me making any additional income.

My partner made enough money to cover most of our bills, but there was little left over for groceries, and we had my infusions to plan around. I looked for small jobs that I could manage, or for things of ours that I could sell, all to keep us solvent. The worst part was not knowing how long it would take to go through the ODSP appeals process, Or whether at the end of the process I would walk away with a judgment in my favor.

In the meantime, the stress negatively impacted my health, prolonging and exacerbating my incapacity.

While struggling to find solutions to the gaps in our budget, there was also a fear about the prospect of making too much money. At what point would Trillium decide that I can afford to pay $10,000 every six weeks? If I managed to get disability and then went back to work, at what point would they decide that I make enough that they no longer have to help provide me with insurance for things like eye care and dental.

I also worried about trying to start a business for fear that welfare would decide that they don't need to help me. After all, I wouldn't need welfare or disability if I was working, right? Ignoring of course that even if I did start a business it could be months before I saw even so much as a penny in profit. Starting a business meant that I might be able to make money after some period of time, and yet I knew doing so might prevent me from getting the financial support I then needed.

In essence, I had to put any plans I might have to claw my way out of poverty on hold or risk losing my chance at getting financial support, thus prolonging the amount of time that I spent financially insecure.

39 Get a Job!

Even if it weren't a matter of being too sick to work, finding a job when you are disabled is incredibly difficult. Any job that requires standing for long periods of time, heavy lifting, or bending can be automatically discounted. There are few options left.

When employers find out that you have Crohn's, as they invariably will either during the interview itself or once you start working, there is a lot of resentment. They don't want to deal with the liability that you represent. When there is a glut of people looking for work, why should they work to accommodate you when they can simply hire someone healthier instead? Even those who are willing to take a chance on you have no concept of how much your condition can affect your ability to work. How can you explain to them how variable your productivity level will be? How can you explain that you are finding it difficult to focus or concentrate, even though you don't look outwardly sick? How can you explain that a condition that doesn't affect anyone else in the office is the reason you have to call in sick as often as you do? How do you explain that you have a legitimate reason to disappear in the bathroom for an hour, or go as often as five, six, or seven times in the morning?

If you get hired during a low-symptom time, it can be difficult to explain to someone why, once hired, you seem to suddenly become very sick, to be admitted for an extended hospital stay, to be in constant pain. And, no, you don't know when it will get better, or even if it ever will. Often, when these observations are made, some well-meaning individual will pop up saying that there are laws protecting people with disabilities; that an employer cannot choose not to hire you because you are disabled. This is true. There are affirmative action policies and laws in place to protect the rights of people with disabilities. The problem is, how do you prove it? How do you prove that you weren't hired due to your disability? No one is going to come out and say, "Yeah, we decided that we don't want to risk working with someone as sick as you" or "We don't want to spend money making this workplace accessible." The employers themselves may not even be fully aware that that is why they didn't hire you.

Many people associate disability or illness with incompetence. This comes from the "just world" fallacy that permeates our culture. We cannot grasp that people can have something bad happen to them without having earned it in some way. We cannot wrap our minds around the idea that someone can be so disproportionately disadvantaged, and so we assume that they must be doing something wrong to have made things difficult for themselves. We see this in how people react to the disproportionate rates of poverty and imprisonment among people of color, how people react to rape and harassment, and so forth. Many people assume that because they have experienced and overcome some form of hardship—as we all do from time to time—that everyone's obstacles must be just as surmountable if they are just willing to tighten their belts, or make healthier lifestyle choices. If only they were willing to make the necessary changes to their lives, they could fix their situations.

It is a blindness that ignores that not all obstacles are the same, and that, in many ways, some obstacles are created and reinforced in our societies in ways that can make them nearly impossible to defeat.

I've mentioned the idea of inspiration porn before and the damage that it can cause, but here in particular we can see its deleterious effects. Inspiration porn, or the prevalence of "success stories," serves as a patina that masks the very real difficulty of these obstacles. It is not that we shouldn't celebrate those successes, but, rather, that those successes shouldn't be used to undermine the difficulties faced by many other people in the same situation. It creates a culture that assumes that anyone who is struggling is incompetent, lazy, or a failure in some way.

When these kinds of thoughts occupy the social mind, it is not surprising that these attitudes pollute how interviewers view us.

40 Start a Business

When people complain about the state of the job market or the difficulty in finding work that fits within their capabilities, many well-meaning people will tell them to start their own business. While the advice has a lot to recommend it in theory, it ignores many of the realities of starting a business.

To start with, you have to have an idea. You can't start a business without some concept of what service or product you would be providing. If most of your experience is as an employee, it can be even more difficult to find an applicable business idea, since your tasks may have already been optimized as much as possible and so problems looking for new solutions might be outside your experience.

Even if you do have a viable idea, starting up is not that easy. No matter what you are doing, there is need for some form of initial financial investment. A financial investment can mean anything from marketing, like website costs, to being able to live without an income until your business starts making money. It takes time—sometimes a long time—for a business to start bringing in enough money to live on. In order to make starting a business financially feasible, you have to be starting from a relatively safe financial place.

If you have ever read financial advice books, many of them often talk about the need to take risks. Authors will often cite their own failed businesses and the money they lost. Frequently, they will make it seem like the consequences of failure are tough but ultimately no big deal. What many of these books ignore is that they themselves already started from a relative place of privilege. They had resources at their disposal, or existed as part of a class that would be given the opportunity to try. Failure might mean debt, but how often did it mean homelessness? How often did it mean the possibility of having to survive without life-saving medication? There is a difference between living poor and living desperate.

Another concern is where you are starting from. I am thinking now of someone struggling with a disability or illness. If you are in the middle of a flare-up, you do not have the energy to devote to developing a new business. It can be difficult just to take care of yourself, let alone devote the umpteen hours a day you need to get a business going.

41 Budget Better

One of the most common bits of advice offered to anyone struggling with poverty is to cut out nonessential expenses. It assumes that people are only poor because they do not know how to manage their money. It assumes that poor people actually do have money, but that they spend it on trivial, inconsequential things that drain their resources. It plays into our societal concept of income being an indicator of intelligence. If they were just a little *smarter*, they wouldn't be so *poor*.

What this advice blatantly ignores is that people who are actually poor don't lack money because they spend too much of it, but rather because they never had it in the first place. If your monthly pay barely covers your rent, you are not going to spend it on useless items. The tendency to spend money beyond what you make, or to waste money on trivialities, is more frequently found among the middle class, not the poor. In order to spend money, you must first have it.

People who struggle from month to month are often much better at budgeting and at knowing how much money they have available than those who don't. Since my financial troubles started, for example, I have known at any given moment the amount of money available in any of my accounts within a few dollars. I have also known exactly where each of those dollars will be applied, whether to rent, groceries, gas, or some other expense. Each purchase is made after running a cost-benefit analysis in my head. Will I get more from this bunch of leeks or from that package of noodles? How many different meals can I make with this bag of rice? How long can I subsist on pasta? People who struggle with money learn to make due with significantly less money than those in higher economic categories.

Having little money means living at the brink of financial insolvency. You need money to be able to save money. The most obvious example of this is when it comes to grocery shopping. A standard bag of pasta costs about $2 in Canada. A bulk bag of pasta contains four times the amount and costs $5. No brainer, right? But what if you only have $3? Should you starve for two weeks till you have enough, or do you buy the smaller bag knowing that you will be paying more in the long run? Bulk stores have upfront membership costs. When it comes to cars, an old car might seem like a more affordable expense until you realize that you pay more in the long run for repairs and poor gas efficiency.

At every turn, money-saving initiatives are reserved for those who have money to begin with.

Sometimes living within your means can mean making financially unsound decisions. Take insurance, for example. Anyone who has gone through a tragedy like their house burning down, as I have, will tell you that having rental insurance (also called tenant insurance) is essential. Without it, you leave yourself at the whim of every natural disaster, of every accident, of every neighbor's unsafe habit. My own home burned down in 2011 and I lost everything because a neighbor's stove malfunctioned. Because I had tenant insurance, I was quickly able to move into a new home and replace some small percentage of what I had lost. Insurance never truly covers everything and so, even years later, I have very few clothes and even fewer extraneous possessions. Most of my furniture I was able to get for free by finding it curbside when students move out of their school-year apartments to either new housing or back home with their parents.

Yet after the coverage that I was eligible for under my parent's home insurance expired, my financial situation made it impossible for me to pay for my own coverage. Every fire alarm leaves me cold with dread as I wonder if this time I will find myself homeless. Without insurance, I wouldn't have the money for a new rent deposit. I don't have the money to buy clothes, furniture, or other necessities that have been lost in a disaster. If there is another fire, it will be a blow from which I might never fully recover.

The advice about cutting out nonessential expenses also ignores that what is essential might change from person to person. In a big city, a car might be deemed unneeded. But what if you work at the other end of town? What if walking is difficult for you, but you have to travel from doctor's appointment to doctor's appointment?

You might think that having a pet is nonessential, but what about studies that show that pet ownership reduces stress? If someone is dealing with a condition that is exacerbated by stress, then having a pet can go a long way toward managing symptoms. Pets are also very effective in helping manage generalized anxiety and symptoms of depression that may be triggered by loneliness. But even more basic, pets are a source of love and affection, something that everyone is entitled to regardless of socioeconomic status. When you claim that poor people should not have pets, you are in essence saying that they are not worthy of love and companionship. What's more, you may be denying that animal a loving and caring home.

What is considered essential or nonessential is not a constant and can change from person to person. Just because you can function without something does not mean that it is the same for everyone. In expecting everyone to conform to your idea of essentiality, you are ignoring the reality that needs differ from person to person.

This type of judgment becomes very apparent in discussions of what qualifies as a "real" poor person. Often this discussion involves examples of people who use their food stamps to buy steak, or some other product that is deemed too highbrow for the lower classes. It is an argument from entitlement which suggests that, in order to have real poverty credibility, you must have the worst of everything—the worst nutrition, the worst living conditions, the worst appearance, and so on. Ignoring the fact that even higher-quality items go on sale from time to time, the argument stems from a need to feel superior. It comes from a need to show that you are better than someone. Even if you are not well-off and will never be rich, at least you are better off, more educated, better dressed, better nourished— just better—than those *poor* people. More than that, this attitude also stems from a desperate desire not to have to face the reality that your "better" status comes from luck as much as anything else—that you could have just as easily been born into a more desperate situation and be facing the same hardships.

Owning up to your privilege is difficult. Doing so, acknowledging that your better position was not earned or deserved in anyway, means acknowledging that we live in an unfair society that privileges some people more than others. Worse than that, it means that even while you benefit from your own privilege, you might be adding and supporting a system of oppression. It forces you to realize that your benefits are supported by the suffering of others. No one likes facing up to the reality that their good might be causing someone else's bad, that they are indirectly responsible for someone else's hardship. It is much easier to blame those who are suffering for their own misfortune. It is much easier to pretend that your success is completely your own creation and not the result of an unfair institution.

This is not to say that those existing at the middle or upper ends of society have never earned anything or are not deserving of praise. To claim so would be to ignore reality just as much as the misguided statements made about the poor. What I mean in all this is that it is important that people be aware of how essential luck is to their success and acknowledge that there is no such thing as an entirely self-made man (or woman, or agender person, or bigender person).

42 Rags to Riches

I want to take a moment to examine the classic rags-to-riches story.

Let us start with a young man who grew up in the projects of some major city. Let us assume that he comes from an immigrant family where English is not spoken at home. To add further hardship, let us assume that he comes from a single-parent home, is the older son, and has several siblings. He is forced to work while going to school to help support his family. He works construction, usually responsible for the most menial tasks on the job site. One day the supervisor notices that his section always manages to have the least amount of accidents or wasted material. The supervisor decides to take a chance on the kid and makes him his assistant. He is responsible for managing one section of the job site and making sure that they have enough supplies to complete the tasks. The kid shines, revealing hidden organizational skills. Soon, he is able to come up with some ideas that save his employer time, money, and frustration. The supervisor recommends him to his boss, and the kid is made a full supervisor on another job site.

Over the next several months, the kid graduates from high school and takes on a full-time position within the company. He is now a supervisor with his own team, working various building projects. Over time, he earns the distinction of having the best-managed sites. In fact, the kid catches potentially fatal mistakes on designs from time to time. His attention to detail and organizational skills impress the company owner, who realizes that the kid has potential to be a great asset to his company. He encourages the kid to take some night business classes at the local community college, and works around his school schedule to make sure he can graduate. When he finishes, the owner gives the kid a high-ranking position within the company, managing several job sites and working as project manager. He runs not just one team but many of them, with many supervisors reporting directly to him.

As the next few years go by, he notices several flaws with how the company is run. He suggests a few improvements, some of which are implemented, while others are ignored. He keeps track of his ideas, as well as making sure to learn as much as he can about running the company. He builds relationships with the clients, earning their admiration and trust.

Finally, he decides to take a chance and start his own competing construction company. He convinces a couple of his employees to join him. He also convinces one of the clients he worked with to give him an opportunity to work on one of their projects. His family scrounges together some money to help him launch. The project is a big success. In the next several years, his company becomes the number one construction company in the city. In fact, his workload has grown so much that he has outright bought the company he used to work for. His managerial style and ideas become the standard in the industry.

He uses some of the money he is making to invest in some building projects of his own and starts making money through real estate as well. He uses his profits to invest in various industries, not tying himself to just one branch of the economy. When trouble hits one industry, he is able to support some of his endeavours through the earnings of other ones. He gets a feel for the market and knows when to sell one of his popular companies and when to buy other struggling ones and turn them around. He is now one of the richest men in his country, through his hard work and dedication. He is a self-made man, making further millions selling his bootstraps story and teaching others how to be as wealthy and successful as he is. Self-made man! But is he really?

It is true that he worked hard. It is true that he overcame hardship and was able to achieve the kind of success that many people only dream of. He had great ideas and great dedication. This is all true and should be celebrated and rewarded. However, to assume that he is a self-made man who achieved all this on his own is simply untrue.

No matter how intelligent this young man was, he would never have been able to get the education he needed unless he lived in a country that provided him with the basics of education in a public institution. If his parents had stayed in their original country, he may not have been afforded the same opportunities, or may have been pushed in a different direction. If his supervisor had not decided to take a chance on him, he could have spent the rest of his life hammering nails. Similarly, his company could have refused to work around his school schedule. They could have made him decide between education and work, a decision that would have impacted his whole family.

His family could have been unwilling to risk their own financial security in order to invest in his endeavour. His first clients could have decided not to risk hiring a new and inexperienced company and gone with the one they had worked with successfully in the past. His friends and employees could have decided not to risk their own security in order to join in on the ground floor of his new venture. He could have had the bad luck to get injured on the job site and become unable to work. He could have been born with a congenital or inherited disability that prevented him from being able to take a physically demanding construction job.

For many people, these are not just hypotheticals. For every successful "self-made man" out there, there are many more who were never afforded the same opportunities, whose businesses failed through no fault of their own, who were never given the opportunity to improve themselves, who may have been forced to choose between completing school and supporting their families, who may have been permanently injured and unable to work, who may have lived in an area with limited opportunities to work for young adults, who may have lived in an area where people of their ethnic background were discriminated against and thus subjected to harassment from teachers, police, and other authority figures. Any of these events could affect the ability of a person to succeed regardless of their dedication and hard work. Luck is a big aspect of success.

Another success story that is often shared is of the amazing person with a disability who manages to gain fame or prosperity: the blind girl who becomes an Olympic athlete, or the deaf person who becomes a world-renowned professor. These stories are impressive and worthy of attention, but not without acknowledging that that blind girl might never have achieved her goals if her parents had not been able to afford to pay for her to do sports or to send her to specialized training. That the professor would never have been able to go to university and earn her degree if there hadn't been support in place to make it possible for her to get an education—if institutions had not been willing to work with her to make learning possible rather than simply lumping her in with the other students and expecting her to fend for herself.

In every success story, it is the support of the community and those around the protagonist that ultimately help make the difference between hard work and success, and hard work and failure. By acknowledging our privilege, we are more likely to help set ourselves up as allies and to provide the support needed to make a difference. When people blind themselves to how others have helped them, to their own luck and privilege, they have to protect that illusion. In order to maintain that narrative, they might refuse to pay it forward, telling others that they need to make it on their own, just like they did.

43 Relationships

The "just world" fallacy affects more than just how the world views those with disability and chronic illnesses; it can also affect how we see ourselves. Although on a conscious level we know that we didn't do anything to deserve this, many of us experience a feeling of being somehow deeply flawed or damaged. Our pain and suffering makes us worth less, somehow, than healthier people.

This idea is reinforced all around us on a daily basis. One tragic example is in how the media portrays us when our parents murder us. When any other child is slain by their parents, it is seen as a tragedy. The parents are condemned as monstrous, as being despicable and without a saving grace. There is a public outcry for them to be punished.

When a parent kills their disabled child, however, there is no public outcry. Instead people trip over themselves to offer explanations and condolences. We were too great a burden. There was not enough support for those poor brave parents. They were overwhelmed. Any excuse justifying why. Even though the result was very sad, it was okay to kill us. The media dehumanizes us. We are not individuals with our own agency, feelings, dreams, hopes, desires. We are burdens, difficulties, accidents, things to be tolerated but not loved and never valued above or as equal to the able-bodied. Our murder is not the action of criminals, but rather a final act of desperation. Poor, poor, parents.

When our murders are painted as acts of desperation rather than crimes, is it surprising that many people with disabilities can fall into the trap of seeing themselves as lesser? Society tells us all the time that we are burdens on everyone else, so why shouldn't we see ourselves that way? Of course that type of thinking can have some very serious repercussions in the relationships that we form with others—with partners, with friends, with family, even with coworkers. If we don't fully acknowledge ourselves as being worthy, it is difficult to expect or enforce that others treat us that way.

If you don't think you are worthwhile, if you think that you are broken and a burden, if you think that no one would want the trouble of being with you, it can be very easy to fall victim to abusive relationships. Emotional abusers in particular prey on vulnerability: "No one else would love you," "No one else would be willing to put up with you the way I do," "No one else would support you the way I do."

In the case of parental or custodial relationships, the caregiver could feel entitled, as though taking care of you or dealing with your disability gives them special privileges or access. They might decide that you owe them for providing you with the means to survive or to function. "I paid for your lifesaving medication, so you owe me." This sense of entitlement can translate into a feeling that they have a right to control you and the life you might not have without the help they've provided; that they get to decide who you marry, where you live, what you study, anything.

Since they spent all that time making sure you got to live, you sure as hell need to make a lot of money so that it was worth it for them. Because of the residual feelings of guilt felt by people who struggle with illness and disability, it can be difficult to fight against that sense of entitlement. In a lot of cases, children feel as though they owe their parents something. "They paid for my medication; it would be ungrateful to cut them out of my life completely even if they are hurting me." This cycle of guilt and shame is self-perpetuating with the abuser feeding off the guilt and using it to shame the victim further: "You are being ungrateful. How dare you expect me to apologize for treating you badly?! I am sorry. Sorry I paid for your medication as long as I did."

The end goal is to wear away further at their self-esteem until the abuser can gain complete control over their victim. They can then use their victim to bolster their own self-esteem about what a good person they are; about how they took such good care of the poor little cripple, how much they sacrificed to do so. Since society tends to side with the caregiver in this situation, it can be extremely difficult for the victim to escape.

The same risk exists in romantic relationships as well. It can be easy to undervalue yourself, to feel as though you are not worthy of a relationship or happiness. While we might talk from time to time about the partner who leaves their sick spouse, we rarely discuss the sick spouse who might want to leave their partner. The assumption is that there is no way that someone who is sick or disabled would be willing or even *want* to leave their romantic partners. After all, they are burdens and should be grateful for the partner who is willing to put up with them. Why would they risk ever finding another who would take someone who comes with so many complications? There can be a lot of pressure, both external and internal, to stay in an unhappy relationship.

Moreover, it can be difficult for the disabled partner to leave. Chances are they are financially dependent on the person they are with. They may be socially isolated and have no support systems available to them outside the home. Disabled partners are more likely to be victims of abuse, both physical and emotional, and their ability to leave may be curtailed not just in the usual ways of abusers, but also by their own bodies as well. What chance has the man in a wheelchair of leaving, if all the exits from the home have stairs? Or what about the bed-ridden patient?

What is important to note, however, is that for all the societal pressure to feel bad about ourselves, the majority of people with disabilities don't actually feel pathetic. We are like anyone else, having our moments of confidence and our moments of self-consciousness. Despite all that, however, we deal with increased pressure and judgment, which can undermine our confidence. It can make it difficult to make the decision that benefits us rather than the one that society expects of us. There is more pressure to play it safe, and to not aim too high.

Moreover, those of us struggling with depression and other mental health issues may have our conditions wreak havoc on our ability to tell healthy situations from unhealthy ones. When your own brain whispers poison in your ear, it can be harder to recognize the venom spewing from other sources.

44 Sex and Dating

The prevailing myth in our culture is that sex and dating is meant for those who are attractive. If you do not cater to the opposite sex by conforming to a strict standard of beauty and health, then you must not be interested in a relationship. Our world desexualizes people with disabilities—so much so that the idea that people with chronic illnesses and disabilities being interested in sex comes as a surprise to many. People who are interested in us are called devotees and are considered fetishists since it is assumed that anyone who is interested in us must be strange or a pervert. This desexualization can make us invisible when it comes to dating culture.

Many discussions of the ethics of sex—whether about consent or safety—often hinge on the ability of those having the discussion to spin a certain behavior as being sexy. So integral is sexiness to our culture that everything from beer to tampons are marketed by appealing to that impulse. The implication is that sexiness equals good sex. It is a concept that does not stack up in reality. Sometimes the best sex can be supremely unsexy. For example: something funny happens and you break into giggles. Does that make it bad sex? No! But most people don't consider sex that has silly elements or moments to be sexy. Or what about lazy I-have-to-get-up-early-in-the-morning-but-we're-both-horny-and-won't-be able-to-sleep-until-we-get-off-so-let's-cuddle-and-have-lazy-sex sex? These are the realities of long-term relationships. Sometimes sex isn't sexy, but it can still be incredible.

One of the foundations of the concepts of sexiness is that of spontaneity. This is problematic not only because of issues like consent or the risk of unplanned pregnancy, but also because of the impact that it has on people with disabilities. Sometimes sex takes planning to accommodate pain, limited mobility, treatment schedules, etc. Most people's idea of sex appeal doesn't include discussions of where best to put the pillow to elevate someone without hurting their back or leg. A lot of people assume that sex that involves that level of preparation cannot be good because it is not spontaneous and therefore not sexy. This in turn might stop people from volunteering information that is necessary to their enjoyment. "Just a moment there, love. Do you think we can stop for a second and maybe change positions? You keep pushing my leg above my head and while it was fun for the first five minutes, now my hip is about to dislocate."

This movement away from discussion actually detracts from enjoyment. Discussion allows you to share desires, erogenous zones, and more. It can lead to exploration and the discovery of mutual kinks.

When dealing with a disability, having to bring up your limitations is often terrifying. What if my requests will be a turn-off? What if drawing attention to my defective body will kill the mood? For partners as well, there's a sense of fragility, and the fear that they might accidentally hurt their partner. Sex education courses usually ignore discussions of sex with illness or disability, and there are few resources with tricks and suggestions.

Some Quick Tips on How to Have Sex with a Disability

It is important that you have some concept of your comfort level and capabilities prior to engaging in sex. Once excited and aroused, it can be easy to get carried away. The pain-minimizing effects of the various hormones can make it easy to go overboard and really hurt yourself. While it may be tempting to try to increase your range of motion through the physical exercise, it is imperative that you don't go so far that you damage yourself further.

Communication Is Essential. If something feels uncomfortable, or if you need to change positions, speak up. Talk to your partner about how to ensure both of you experience pleasure. You might want to discuss toys that can be brought in, or different forms of sexual expression that might be easier for you. While it is important to communicate during sex, it is even more important to have these discussions before you become intimate. A discussion now can save embarrassment and frustration later.

Relax. One of the quickest ways to get in the way of good sex is to worry too much. Don't place too much value on every time being perfect, or on meeting some impossible standard. Sex, even when it goes wrong, can be an enjoyable experience. If part of your body is not cooperating at any given moment, try something different. Oral sex, mutual masturbation, and frottage are all sex.

Enjoy touching one another. Find pleasure in different forms of touch, from soft and sensitive, to more intense. Make each physical interaction, like a hug or even a pat on the back, a special one and learn to appreciate them fully. Appreciate them in the moment, not just for what they can lead to. Enjoy the sensuality of a massage, for example, without the pressure of it being a prelude to something else. Explore your body and your partner's body, and take pleasure in both.

Support Yourself. Using pillows for support and as a shock absorber can minimize a lot of problems when having sex. You can use them to prop up your back, legs, arms, and other parts of your body. You can also use furniture to help facilitate different positions. For example, if you like being on top but can't bend your knees too much or put weight on your knees, have your partner sit on a chair that lets you be on top of them, but with your knees straighter. Use your feet and the floor to help make the necessary up and down motions.

Supporting yourself can also mean planning sex in ways that work better with your body. If you find yourself to be in a great deal of pain after eating, try having sex before meals! If you get really tired in the evenings, or are really stiff in the mornings, plan around those times. Sometimes sex can actually be used to help you lower your symptoms. If that is the case, don't feel guilty or ashamed for doing so. Sex can be a great muscle relaxant and painkiller!

Practice Self-care and Encourage Your Partner to Do the Same. If you need to take a break during sex because you are too sore or too tired, do so. If you need to spend the next twenty minutes after sex winding down or letting your energy regenerate, do so. If you need your partner to rub your leg after sex to help with blood flow, talk about it and work out a fair compromise to make it possible for them to do so. The more you take care of yourself surrounding issues of sex, the more willing and receptive to sexual activity you will be.

Of course, all this assumes you are interested in sex. If you don't have sexual urges, or have an asexual orientation, that is okay too. Just be honest with yourself and with your partner. You are not responsible for defending the sexuality of people with disabilities by doing something you yourself don't want to do.

There are lots of different disabilities and it would be impossible to give specific advice for each one, especially not in a book about a different topic. The most important advice I can leave you with, however, is to work within your own comfort level and explore your limits. Find out what works for you and work it! Remember also that different bodies work differently and that there is no "right way" to orgasm. Many people find that their specific disabilities change how they experience touch, desire, etc. For example, people with spinal injuries may have limited sensation in their genitals, but increased sensitivity somewhere else. They may require more intense stimulation of the genitalia, or they may need a different part of their body to be stimulated.

Neither sex ed nor doctors often discuss the effects of disability, injury, and even surgery on one's ability to experience and enjoy sex. As a result, many patients may be faced with an arduous process of discovery, or may become discouraged and believe that they are incapable of sexual pleasure. There needs to be more research and more time devoted to sexual studies of the disabled, so that patients don't get left behind because of social assumptions.

For partners of people with disabilities, it can be difficult to know how to behave in terms of sexual interaction. You might want to initiate but worry about pushing them too far or pressuring them into something they are unwilling or unable to do at that time. This fear can lead partners to avoid initiation, which can backfire by making the person with a disability question whether their partner finds them attractive.

It can be difficult to navigate the situation, and that is understandable. There is truth in the advice that you should treat them as a human being, giving them the same autonomy, respect, and individuality that you would anyone else. It is also true that there are also very real considerations to keep in mind, especially in relation to how our culture paints disability sexuality.

One important bit of advice is to trust your partner. If they say they are okay, trust them. Ironically enough, being overly concerned about whether or not they are really able to do something, about whether or not they are in pain, can actually put them at more risk than if you simply trust them. They, we, might feel the need to overcompensate in order to put you at ease. If someone is always worrying about me, it makes it difficult to be honest when I really do need help, or when I really cannot do something. There is a fear that being honest in those situations might reinforce the idea of my helplessness in their mind. If my partner, on the other hand, trusts me to be honest with them about when I am fine, then I feel more comfortable being honest with them about when I am not. I don't feel like I always have to prove that I am productive, that I am not helpless, and that I am capable. I can trust them to know that there are moments when I am vulnerable and incapable of doing something, but that that doesn't affect my ability in other ways or on other days.

Another important consideration is to not guilt or shame your partner for not being sexually available or incapable of certain things. While it can be frustrating to have your ability to have frequent sex curtailed by something like your partner's frequent fatigue and pain, remember that you are not the only one affected by it. In fact, it is important to remember that your partner is not just dealing with pain and fatigue, but may also be dealing with their own sexual frustration as well. Statements like, "Oh great, you are tired again!" or "You were able to lift your leg this morning when you went to work!" or "My last girlfriend was able to do ____!" are damaging and can make your partner even more reluctant to engage in sexual activity. While it is true that prolonged dry spells due to health constraints can impact your own psychological health—such as damaging your own self-esteem and perception of your attractiveness—there are better ways to discuss these issues than by employing shaming techniques.

Instead of blaming your partner for their inability to engage in sexual activity, discuss your concerns from a personal perspective. Instead of "You never want to have sex anymore!" try "I know you are feeling sick and cannot have sex as often or the way we did before, but I am starting to feel unappreciated and unattractive. Perhaps we can come up with low-energy compromises that would keep the intimacy in our relationship?" Just as it is important for people with disabilities to remember that things like oral sex and frottage count as sex, so too is it important for their partners to remember the same as well. If you do manage to come up with a compromise, remember not to complain about the outcome. If you are complaining about how oral sex is not real sex, then it can drain the desire for your partner to try for a compromise.

The compromise does not always mean engaging in sexual activity. It can mean your partner making an effort to show you affection and intimacy in ways that are within their capabilities at that time. This may mean more frequent comments or compliments about your attractiveness, more cuddles, more hugs, and so forth. Many times, people who are struggling with their pain and fatigue and are unable to offer the level of sexual contact that you might desire already feel guilty on their own. They might be looking for a way to bring up their concerns without putting their guilt over on you instead.

It is important in any relationship to maintain open and honest communication. By bringing up concerns as they come up, you reduce the likelihood that they will become problems or resentments later on. By being open and honest with one another, you might notice that your concerns are very similar. By maintaining communication, it can be easier to come up with solutions and compromises since you are not just suddenly trying to come up with ideas without ever having considered the subject. Similarly it means that you aren't trying to come up with ideas having never discussed sex previously.

Another suggestion that might help partners is to help minimize their symptoms. Since a lot of what gets in the way of intimacy and activity is fatigue and pain, helping to reduce those might increase sexual frequency. This can include providing massages, administering warm compresses, or taking over some of their regular chores and responsibilities. The easiest way to know what you can do to help is to ask. There is that communication again.

45 Depression and Doctors

When struggling with pain, constant fatigue, nausea, malnutrition, loneliness, and a variety of other symptoms, it is common for people dealing with chronic illness and disability to be vulnerable to depression. It could be that you are simply overwhelmed by situations caused or worsened by your condition, such as the stress of managing symptoms, nutrient deficiencies caused by an inability to properly digest your food, or an inability to practice adequate self-care.

With all the concern about managing your apparently more serious chronic symptoms, it can be tempting to simply ignore your mental health. It makes sense that you are depressed. Who wouldn't be if they lived like you? You already have all these other drugs, do you really need to add antidepressants? It's not like you are going to hurt yourself, you don't have the energy. And even if you did, would anyone care? You would stop being a burden. No one would have to worry about you anymore. It would stop the pain . . .

Just like that, the depression becomes severe and cause for concern. At the worst moments during a flare, you might be stuck indoors for long periods of time alone. You might be in a hospital bed, your only human interaction with nurses and, perhaps, the occasional visitor. You wake up to the touch of someone there to take your blood each morning, and this may be your day's longest physical contact.

Regardless of whether you see a lot of people or none at all, you are stuck in one place for a long time. Imagine having to spend the entire day in a small, somewhat uncomfortable bed. The only time you get up is to go to the bathroom, and to do that you have to push the IV pole attached to your arm.

Even if you aren't hospitalized, the exhaustion can create the same results at home. After a while it starts to drain you even further. Your life starts to stretch out before you, an endless miasma of pain and boredom. You don't even have the energy to watch TV. You just want to lie in bed and wish you could find the energy to have a shower.

It can further complicate the situation that symptoms of many chronic conditions and depression often overlap: fatigue, difficulty falling asleep, lack of energy, pain, and so forth. It can be difficult to tell when you are dealing with one thing or another. Are you unable to get motivated because your Crohn's kept you up all night, or because your depression is making it hard to care about anything? Is the exhaustion mental or physical? Is my joint pain a physical response to inflammation or to psychological pain? Moreover, sometimes physical pain can cause the psychological pain. It all intertwines until it is almost impossible to tell.

Despite the frequent connection between disabilities, illnesses, and anxiety/depressive disorders, the medical community still has a hard time understanding the correlation. Frequently a psychological diagnosis is treated very negatively. Even if you have a documented disorder that you are being treated for, a diagnosis of any psychological condition could mean a decrease in the quality of care. Suddenly, every trip to the doctor or ER becomes suspect. Some doctors will wonder if you are faking your symptoms in order to score drugs, while others will assume you are overreacting or confusing mental symptoms with physical ones. It creates a situation where there is an incentive for people with chronic conditions not to seek help for their related psychological conditions.

I have seen this manifest personally. The usual procedure when I come into the hospital is to be given an antinausea agent and pain medications. Regardless of whether they think I need to be admitted or not, the usual assumption is that if the pain is bad enough for me to feel the need to come in, then controlling the pain is a concern. On one such occasion, I noticed a slight change in how I was treated. Usually there is an effort to reduce my pain symptoms as quickly as possible. This time around, it seemed that there was a hesitancy to do anything about it. I was offered some antinausea medication, but not once was there even a mention of anything to do about the pain.

When the doctor came in to see me, the first questions were not about why I was there, but clarifications about my last visit to the hospital being labeled "psychiatric." I was confused, having never come to the hospital for anything mental-health related. I racked my brain for every time I had been to the hospital in the last few months: visit with my gastroenterologist, visit with my rheumatologist, weight management clinic . . . Bingo. It seems that the clinic I had visited to see about getting help in losing weight with the difficulty of Crohn's and arthritis registered as a psychiatric visit on my hospital file.

In combination with my medication for anxiety, depression, and ADHD, they had assumed that I had come in to be treated for something else. The pallor of having sought help for a mental-health problem changed how they viewed my physical health. I never was offered anything for pain, and I was sent home without any satisfactory aid for what was wrong with me. For the first time I was given the answer that it was "just Crohn's." A condition that had such a profound impact on my life was suddenly seen as no big deal because of one tick on my chart that might suggest that I also had a psychiatric disorder, in this case depression. That the Crohn's might be the cause of the depression was never considered. That a person can have two things wrong with them and have them be equally valid and serious was never considered. No, despite the fact that I had a documented physical condition, my depression, anxiety, and any other mental-health disorder I might have meant that the pain was all in my head.

46 Paging Dr. Feminist

This idea that emotional health somehow impacts the validity of physical concerns is often seen in the bias that many medical professionals hold toward women. In many cases, women have a harder time having their concerns taken seriously by doctors due to the assumption that they were somehow hysterical and were exaggerating the pain.

It is not difficult to find multiple examples of doctors dismissing as cramps a woman's concerns about abdominal pain near her ovaries that later revealed an ovarian cyst or tumor. It is also common for iron-deficiency anemia in women to be dismissed as being caused by menstrual bleeding. I have long had low blood iron scores, only to be told that I don't eat enough meat and that my period is making it worse. One of the reasons I started taking birth control pills was to reduce my anemia. Years later, when birth control pills weren't helping, my case was found to follow the pattern revealed in recent studies: that iron deficiency in women is caused not by menstruation, but often by gastrointestinal bleedsing If doctors had taken the time to investigate why I was anemic, it is possible that I would have received a Crohn's diagnosis long before the symptoms made themselves felt as strongly as they did. It is possible that it would have been discovered while it was still mild enough to be treated with less severe medication.

There are endless stories of people whose health and treatment were affected by negative gender stereotypes. When talking to men struggling with mental-health issues, it is not uncommon to hear that they have been mocked for having a "woman's complaint." Often depression, eating disorders, anxiety, and other such concerns are stigmatized as being weak or woman-like; that mental-health complaints are nothing more than emotionality. It falls into the idea that "emotionality" is the domain of the "weaker" sex and is not a real concern. Frequently, people with depression are told to just "get over it" or "quit complaining." Men who dare to admit to any of these conditions are made to feel ashamed not just for the fact that they are sick, but also for being a disappointment to their gender.

Alternately, many women find their concerns to be treated with less weight. One story that springs to mind is of another friend with Crohn's: she was recovering at home from major abdominal surgery when a nurse suspected that she might have an air embolism and recommend that she immediately go to the emergency room. While there, the doctor on call chose to believe that she was overreacting and faking it. Even after the nurse came in to explain her concerns, and after being shown her chart and the still healing scar from the surgery, the doctor refused to take the complaint seriously, going so far as to suggest the possibility of her having inflicted the wound on herself. The nurse was flabbergasted at the accusation. Eventually she received treatment, but she was kept in a dangerous state for longer than was safe or necessary. Why? Because women are considered to be unreliable.

Female sufferers of chronic conditions frequently find that the level of pain they must experience before they are taken seriously is significantly higher than that of men with the same condition. This is influenced by the idea that women are weak and deal poorly with pain, and thus are likely to be overreacting. Men, on the other hand, are believed to be tougher. If they come in to have something checked out, it is taken more seriously. What this attitude blatantly ignores is that chronic pain sufferers, regardless of gender, are forced to cope with higher than normal levels of pain on a daily basis. Their tolerance for pain tends to be much higher than the general population. If something is serious enough for them to consider going to the hospital, a process that is exhausting, there is usually something new going on or the pain is particularly strong.

The disparity between the treatment of male and female patients is often believed to be, at least partially, explained by the low prevalence of female doctors and scientists. While there is truth to this, that alone would not fix the situation as even women are not immune to the social bias against women. In addition, medical industries have historically been biased toward male populations as being representative of "typical" presentation, ignoring how female populations may present the same disorders differently.

The severity of this bias came to the fore somewhat recently when it was discovered that women experiencing a heart attack often do not display the usual chest pain and arm numbness symptoms classically associated with that condition. Instead, many women present with stomach upset and general discomfort. In fact, many women presenting with "typical" heart attack symptoms are now thought to have actually experienced milder heart attacks in the past that were not recognized as such. In a recent discussion with my friend Miranda, a nurse in Canada, she mentioned a presentation she had attended by a cardiologist. This presentation included a discussion of how the elderly, those with diabetes, and women all presented with "atypical" symptoms of heart attacks, and the resulting fear this cardiologist had of being faced with an elderly diabetic woman. My question, of course, was if these "atypical" symptoms were being found among such a large population, shouldn't they just be considered the "typical" symptoms? The medical community treats men as the standard of normalcy even when they represent a minority of overall cases.

By using cis men as the standard of normalcy, many studies ignore how medications might interact differently with patients who are not cis men. The standard dose of a medication is often based only on interactions with a cis male body, which means that the same dose taken by a woman may be less effective or may be too much. They may not take into account the interactions between higher levels of certain hormones, or increased body fat content. Even weight-based dosages might ignore that a male-bodied and female-bodied person of the same weight will most likely have different compositions of fat and muscle. If the medication is fat soluble or rendered less effective by the presence of fat, then the female-bodied patient may be receiving the wrong dosage.

For those drugs made specifically for women, the most robust studies of them often focus on how the drugs will impact fetal development, sending the message that the medical field only cares about women insofar as their treatment may impact their pregnancies.

47 Beyond the Chart

Regardless of gender dynamics, there is a necessity for an overall change in attitude in the medical field in general and among doctors in particular. It has been my experience, and that of many other patients, that doctors are so often convinced of their own all-knowingness that they often ignore the patient.

To some extent this is understandable. Doctors spend years studying medicine and have a much greater understanding of many health issues than the lay population. However, in the case of chronic illness, patients become avid students of their own bodies—so much so that we can learn to deduce from the most subtle symptoms an oncoming storm. We learn our bodies out of necessity. We need to know when to avoid certain foods or activities, and when going a bit overboard is okay. We know how medication affects us; we learn what works and what doesn't. We memorize our bodies because it can mean the difference between being functional or bedridden for days. More than anything, we become attuned to what is normal for us and what isn't.

If I come in to the hospital because of abnormal abdominal pain, I am there because something has changed. It might still be Crohn's but it would mean that the Crohn's has moved to a new location or has suddenly worsened; both possibilities are worth investigating. It could also be a new problem manifesting itself.

I remember coming in to the ER once because my pain had somehow shifted. It was not perhaps worse than what I had experienced with Crohn's in the past, but it felt different. Throughout the examination process I was asked again and again if I was sure it wasn't Crohn's. I wasn't, but I also knew that the new pain could mean that I had a blockage, a fistula, or any other variety of complications from Crohn's that would require medical intervention. In order to be taken seriously I had to insist that I was sure it wasn't. Sure enough, it was soon discovered that it was pancreatitis. I needed to be admitted and put on pain medications and a liquid diet.

There is an old adage that says that everything starts to look like a nail when all you have is a hammer. Similarly, when you have a chronic illness, the assumption is that if anything ever goes wrong with you it is directly related to your chronic illness. While it is true that a chronic illness tends to consume your life, it is not a magic barrier preventing you from ever getting sick from something else. Quite the opposite, in fact. By assuming that every problem is related to Crohn's, doctors create a situation where a patient may need to lie—or, at least, fudge the truth a little—to have their symptoms taken seriously.

When your whole life is dictated by pain, you learn everything about it. In some ways, it is a bit like a lover. You learn what makes it tick, you learn to recognize when it is acting out or acting up. You learn the difference between a sharp pain and a throbbing one and what they may indicate. You learn what a sharp pain in spot A means verses a sharp one in spot B. It is next to impossible to communicate that wealth of knowledge to doctors convinced of their own superior knowledge. While it is true that the doctor might be an expert on Crohn's, I am an expert on me. Ignoring the patient's self-knowledge means more work for the doctor in the long run.

The relationship between patients and doctors is becoming increasingly adversarial. Doctors struggle with increasing caseloads, which means less time to spend with patients and more time correcting and addressing misinformation from the Internet and other sources. Patients, on the other hand, are increasingly frustrated with doctor attitudes and lack of time, driving them to the Internet and other sources to get answers, without the training or scientific background to be able to distinguish pseudoscience and conspiracy theories from actual information. The result is a self-perpetuating cycle that ends with frustration and no results.

While it may seem unfair to expect doctors to be the ones to change their behavior when the fault lies on both sides, the expectation stems from the division of power. Doctors have authority and treatments on their side, whereas the patient has fear, pain, and the feeling of not being in control. That fear is rarely addressed in an appointment setting. That fear doesn't go away even when the patient is used to living with a chronic condition.

For all that I am used to going to the ER and being admitted regularly, I am still afraid.

I don't fear doctors, or needles, or even being in the hospital. Rather, I fear always being in pain, needing surgery, losing even more independence than I already have. Each trip to the hospital could mean something new. It could mean that my condition has gotten worse or that I have a brand new diagnosis to live with. Each trip means the possibility of surgery. Each trip means the possibility of new drugs, which means having to struggle through administrative hurdles yet again to be able to get them. It is the fear of the unknown and the known all at once.

I am better at living with that fear than I was, but that doesn't mean the fear has gone away. Having to deal with doctors who treat me like an idiot, or ignore what I am saying, or decide that I must be faking it doesn't help. It adds another fear to the list, so that now each trip is accompanied with the question: "Will I be believed? Or have I been here one time too many? Am I going to be treated like a patient or a criminal? Like someone in pain, or like a drug seeker looking to score?"

One of the barriers toward greater understanding between patients and doctors is the fact that many doctors forget that the symptoms they rely on for diagnosis are actual experiences that the patient deals with, not just a word on the page. Moreover, a diagnosis or lack of diagnosis does not make those experiences stop. It is not unheard of for patients with chronic illnesses to leave the hospital feeling worse than when they came in. The major difference being that despite the fact they are feeling worse, their symptoms are back to the "norm" for their conditions. That doesn't necessarily make them any less unpleasant or easier to bear.

For many doctors, the way they go about their exams and tests makes it seem like they forget that the recipient of all of them is a human being. That for every blood test they run, there is a person who is experiencing that needle prick. For every abdominal palpitation, the pain response may be the result of the fact that they are treating the body like it is made of wood with no sensory ability other than the pain that brought them in. I cannot count how often I responded to the feeling of being pierced by someone's fingernail as much as to the fact that the area they were palpitating was sore to begin with.

48 Fat Shaming Hurts

If you are also overweight, the problem escalates further. Weight is never seen as a symptom, always as a cause. There are endless stories of times when doctors ignore potential problems due to their insistence that everything would get better if the patient just lost 20, 30, 40, or 50 pounds. If you are overweight, whether medically or only culturally, every visit starts with a battle just to have them see past the numbers on the scale. Your limited time in the office is taken up with insistence that your diet is good and you exercise sufficiently.

If either of those are not the case, then further time may be eaten up by an explanation of why you aren't able to be the perfect fatty who eats salad and works out X hours a day. The fact that your joints hurt due to a preexisting condition cannot be used as an explanation because even if you have X-rays, tests, and countless other confirmations on your side, your joint pain is always the result of your weight. Your weight is never the result of your joint pain.

Even when dealing with specialists for my conditions, I am often faced with a significant portion of time being dedicated to a discussion of my weight. That this discussion is one that is triggering for me and one that has visible negative consequences on my health is never important. What matters is that the doctors make sure that I understand completely that being on medication that makes me gain weight, having to accommodate my conditions with a diet that is not optimized for weight loss, and being permanently disabled in my hip in a way that makes most exercise impossible, are all not excuses for being aesthetically unpleasing.

When my weight is consistently made a central issue, the "fat blindness" of my doctors becomes the greatest risk my weight poses to my health.

There's a connection between weight shaming and problematic attitudes from medical professionals in other areas, as I learned all to well when I was assaulted by a doctor.

At eighteen, I went to see a doctor at the university clinic to be tested for bacterial vaginosis, a condition in which the natural bacterial population in the genitals are disrupted and begin to grow abnormally. It is characterized by a strong odor, and I was nervous. You see, I was in love and I wanted to make sure that I didn't smell funny or strange if the chance to have sex ever came up.

The doctor I saw for the initial testing was very kind. The condition is diagnosed by a swab, and she opted not to use a speculum because I was a virgin—the same decision made by all doctors I had seen previously for gynecological issues.

A few weeks later, I was called back into the clinic to get my results. For this follow-up appointment, I saw a different doctor. She was tall, slim, and blond. I was there to get my results to find out if I had bacterial vaginosis, but before she even got to those she began lecturing about my weight. She told me I was morbidly obese. She told me that if I was worried about smell, that I probably had diabetes and that that's what I was smelling. I didn't know what fat shaming was then; at least, I hadn't heard the name, only experienced it. I tried standing up for myself, letting her know that I had been tested and that my cholesterol, my blood pressure, and my blood sugar levels were all perfect. I was about forty pounds heavier than the optimal weight for my height.

The facts didn't matter. The doctor decided that I didn't meet her standards of fitness and she decided that the best way to deal with it was to make me feel horrible about myself. When we finally got to the results, she told me that I did not have bacterial vaginosis. She asked me why I had come in to check on it, and so I told her about my insecurities regarding a smell. Unexpectedly, she offered to take a look. I was shocked, but I accepted her offer. I was worried, but she was a doctor. She had to be professional, right?

As I sat on the table, getting ready for the exam, I asked her not to use the speculum. I was a virgin, I told her. I told her the other doctor said it wasn't necessary, and I really preferred that she not use it.

I lay down on the cold table.

It's a vulnerable position. Everything about a doctor's office is about power. You sit, while the doctor stands above you. You are naked, while they are dressed. You are in pain, afraid, vulnerable, and they hold the answers. Everything about the doctor-patient relationship reinforces that power dynamic.

I was vulnerable on that table, exposing myself, my private parts, to a doctor who had already wounded me. She had already established her power over me, so I knew that my request was a supplication. It was her power to grant it. But she didn't.

As I lay there exposed on the cold table, worried about whether or not I was normal, the doctor violated my request. She shoved an unlubricated speculum inside me and opened it to its widest setting. I can't even remember what came next. I do remember the pain, though that was only a small part of what I was feeling.

I don't remember walking out of the clinic, but I do remember walking back to my dorm. I remember rushing, trying to reach privacy before I started crying. I went first to the room of the person I trusted most on campus, but he wasn't there. He wasn't there and in my search for him I ended up in a room with some people I only vaguely knew, but by then it was too late. I broke down crying. I told them what happened. I was bleeding, I was sure of it. I felt torn. But I was crying about the fat shaming. I had every instance I had ever been called fat flying through my brain.

I was lucky in some ways. These people I barely knew, who comforted me as I cried, said all the right things. They told me that what happened was assault, and that it wasn't my fault. That what she had done was wrong and that I was right to be upset. Not everyone is so lucky.

I didn't want to listen. I wasn't prepared to face that what happened to me was assault, so instead I concentrated on the fat shaming. I focused on what she had said prior to the assault, forcing myself to believe that that was what was upsetting me. I convinced myself that the assault was no big deal. I ignored it.

But it wasn't "no big deal." When I lost my virginity years later, I postponed getting a pap smear. Normally, women are encouraged to get one within a year of becoming sexually active, yet I postponed it for two years. I didn't want to be in that vulnerable position again.

Moreover, I became more sensitive to fat shaming. I lost my temper a lot quicker whenever any mention of my weight was made.

That experience tinged all my subsequent interactions with doctors. Whenever doctors decided to bring up my weight, I found it more difficult to trust them or found myself reacting negatively to the rest of the appointment. Every time a doctor failed to listen to me, it felt like another betrayal. I found myself avoiding those doctors and having an aversion to seeing them again.

49 Triggered

Everything came to a head when my GI decided to send me to a weight management clinic. My appointment was in the evening. The morning of the appointment, I woke up in a panic. My heart was beating furiously, I was sweating, I couldn't focus my mind. I found myself sitting in a corner, rocking back and forth, crying. I couldn't understand why.

In discussions of sexual assault, posttraumatic stress disorder (or PTSD), and anxiety, we often talk about triggers. I had a general understanding of what a trigger was, but now I was experiencing one. I was having a panic attack. All I could think about was that doctor, her cold hands, the pain of the rough plastic edges as the speculum entered me, the stretching and tearing as it was being opened. I couldn't get the feeling of betrayal out of my mind, the feeling of being violated. Superimposed over those feelings was every instance a doctor refused to listen to me. When my hip joint was inflamed and my femur slowly being destroyed by illness, the doctor's only concern was that it was not cancer. All the times I had told doctors that I was in pain and was ignored. All the times that I had had to be vulnerable with a doctor and had that vulnerability rewarded with pain and betrayal.

When I realized what was going on, I took some anxiety medication and tried to calm myself down. Even so, I spent the day curled around myself, trying to hold myself together, as I watched the clock tick down to my appointment. I was terrified. I didn't know what would happen when I went into the clinic. Would I be subjected to the same level of shaming? Would these doctors ignore me like so many other doctors had? Would they see me as some project for them to fix rather a human being?

Throughout my struggle, I realized that what I had told myself was no big deal had actually been affecting my interaction with doctors for years.

I had spoken about my assault before in public forums, and while I knew that what the doctor had done was wrong, I insisted that I was okay. What I hadn't realized was how far down I had buried the pain that that assault had caused.

Now suddenly I was being faced with the truth. That what happened to me was a big deal. It was a big fucking deal. I had been assaulted. By a doctor. By a member of society that I was supposed to be able to trust implicitly. By a person that everyone expects me to trust. Not only had my body been violated, so had my ability to trust that doctors were working in my best interests. What's more, the violation brought on the realization that I was very much a member of a vulnerable population. In discussions of sexual assault, we often forget to mention that people with disabilities are among some of the most at risk for sexual assault.

Sexual assault is not about sex, it is about power. It is about the perpetrator feeling like they have power over someone else—the victim. Maybe it is the result of their own feelings of powerlessness. Maybe it comes from some psychopathic instinct that other people don't matter, that only their own feelings matter. I don't know. I do know that the inclusion of my genitals in this assault was incidental. The doctor in question wasn't trying to get any kind of sexual thrill. She wasn't trying to cater to some sexual desire. It had nothing to do with what I was wearing, or how I looked, or anything else about me. It simply came down to her need to feel powerful. I didn't matter. Who I was didn't matter. She just needed to assert her own power over someone else, and I just happened to be the one on her examination table.

If you asked her, she probably would have no idea that what she did to me was assault. She might excuse her actions, saying that the use of a speculum was necessary in my exam. She might defend herself saying that she is a doctor and I am not, and that she knew better than I did.

Others have told me the same thing. Whenever I discuss what happened to me, someone always feels the need to mention that the doctor might not have been thinking about consent but might have simply decided that using a speculum was necessary. They are the ones who know better, after all. Who am I as an untrained patient to decide what equipment a doctor needs or doesn't need?

Just because they know better, does that mean they have a right to ignore the boundaries I set for myself? Does that mean that I have no say in what happens to my body? And if so, is my body really mine? What about your body? And where do we draw the line?

It doesn't matter if the use of the speculum really was the best medical practice—I made my boundaries clear and she violated them. I told her in no uncertain terms what she couldn't do to my body and she ignored me. I said no, but she did it anyway. She inserted an object into my body after I had said no. That is assault, and no question about it.

The fact that she did so without even the courtesy of using lubrication, which is a standard procedure in those types of medical procedures, merely reinforces the malice behind her actions. To her, it didn't matter if I felt pain. I wasn't a human being in that moment. I was a victim. I was at her mercy. She was the one in charge and she could do whatever she wanted to me without fear of consequences. Even if she had used lubrication, it would have made little difference. She inserted an object into me after I had said no. She ignored my no. To her, what I wanted didn't matter. That is what makes it assault.

Whenever people share tips about how to avoid sexual assault, what they are ignoring is that the victim is not the objective of the assault. To the assaulter, the victim is not a person. They are a feeling. Some rapists might have a list of criteria that the victim must meet in order to perfect the feeling for them. Maybe they need to look like someone who makes them feel powerless. Maybe they need to be vulnerable in some way. In the end it doesn't matter. What matters is that the person committing assault chooses to ignore the humanity of their victim in order to assuage some need of their own—a psychological need, not a sexual one. Some need that matters more to the assaulted than the harm they are doing, the pain they are causing to another human being. The assault is not about the victim, it is about the assaulter. Sharing tips for avoiding rape ignores that.

Assaults by doctors, unless sensationalized and existing on a large scale, rarely get talked about. We put great faith in doctors, we elevate them to almost godlike levels, believing them to be pillars of virtue, goodness, and intelligence. We don't want to face that the people responsible for our health and well-being might be as human as the rest of us. We don't want to address the fact that power dynamics that are enforced as severely as those between patients and doctors put us at risk of abuse. We don't want to believe that the old adage about the corrupting influence of power might apply to doctors, too.

We especially don't want to talk about doctor abuse because, in doing so, we risk being lumped in with conspiracy theorists who condemn the medical profession as a whole. As an advocate of evidence-based medicine, how can I draw attention to abuses perpetuated by doctors and still defend them as a profession?

And yet, drawing attention to this abuse is very important. When someone is hurt so personally by a doctor, it can be easy to lose faith in the entire industry. Being violated by a doctor does more than affect you psychologically, it can also put your health at risk. It can make you afraid to be vulnerable with doctors again. It might mean that you don't seek medical treatment when it is necessary, or that you hide a symptom from your doctor.

More importantly, talking about doctor abuse is essential to help victims realize that they didn't do anything wrong and that they are not alone.

50 Religion and Disability

I am often asked what accessibility and disability have to do with atheism and secular activism. In North American culture, religion tends to be seen as a source of comfort and support, particularly in the context of a health crisis. I have often heard that, while religion may not be useful in a medical context, it's at least harmless. I have not found that to be the case, however, and I could not write this book without including at least one chapter on the harm that religion can do with regard to health.

"Just World" Fallacy

I've already mentioned the idea that bad things happen to people for a reason. We desperately want there to be a reason why one person gets sick and another person doesn't. In part, this idea stems from fear, because we don't want to think that bad things could happen to us. But another part of it stems from guilt. If bad things can happen to anyone regardless of merit, then the fact that you are not sick, or haven't had this terrible thing happen to you, is just (or, at least, partially) luck. You didn't do anything to deserve your good fortune, just as they didn't do anything to deserve their misfortune. The impulse toward the "just world" fallacy is understandable, but it can be incredibly damaging to those struggling.

One of the ways in which religion can cause harm for those of us with disabilities is that many—arguably most—codify this fallacy as a tenet of their religious beliefs.

One of the first examples to come to mind is the concept of karma: a philosophical concept that is present in many Eastern-originated religions regarding actions or deeds that fuel the process of cause and effect. A simplistic explanation would be that a cosmic tally of your life's deeds determines your next reincarnation, so that a tally of good deeds leads to reincarnation as something better while a history of misdeeds would cause one to be reincarnated in a less favorable position. It is used to explain why some people are born in poverty while others are born into wealth. It is sometimes misunderstood by people who do not follow those religions as taking place within the same lifetime, so that someone tripping right after neglecting to tip a waitress is thought to be karmic retribution.

Since disability and illness are rarely, if ever, considered positive additions to someone's life, karma is invoked to assume that the individual must have done something to deserve their health troubles. Illness and disability are punishments, and so it would be unfair to mitigate their effects. Doing so would be interfering with cosmic justice.

The idea that disability is deserved is not limited to karmic religions. The faith-healing traditions of many Christian sects, for example, operate on the assumption that disability and illness are sent by God and can be cured only with complete faith and trust in the Lord. Following this belief to its logical conclusion, we might assume that anyone who remains ill or disabled can have only themselves to blame. They didn't believe enough. They did not allow themselves to be healed.

This belief is not unique to fundamentalist churches. Even in more mainstream denominations, people pray to get better and for pain to stop. Doing so comes saddled with the expectation that if they don't get better, they haven't prayed enough, haven't believed enough, or haven't trusted enough to God. It is not always spelled out, and not everyone says or thinks it, but you hear it implied whenever someone says, "I'll pray for you" or "You should pray for a miracle." Even when others' expectations for you are not on your mind, when you are a sick believer, you blame yourself. Why did this happen to me? What did I do to deserve it? What must I do for a miracle? Why am I being punished? Why am I not worth helping or saving?

Mother Teresa and the Ecstasy of Suffering

The world praised Mother Teresa for her service to humanity since well before her death. Yet we have now seen the publication of several books and studies showing that the praise she has received may have been unwarranted. Her organization raised millions, perhaps even billions, of dollars—certainly enough to build a state-of-the-art hospital that could have either cured, treated, or at least made comfortable the suffering to which she tended.

Instead, Mother Teresa spoke out about the blessedness of suffering. Suffering brings us closer to God, she said, because the suffering of the sick mimics Christ's suffering on the cross. In the minds of many Catholics, and other Christian sects as well, suffering confers a type of holiness. While it may seem nice, perhaps beneficial, to so elevate the status of those who suffer, in reality it can be just as damaging as the idea that suffering is deserved.

When suffering is elevated to a state of holiness, there is little reason to lessen it. People stop seeing prolonged suffering as something that is happening to people, but rather as a sort of sacrament. If suffering isn't something that happens to people, to human beings, but rather happens to inspirational objects, then accessibility doesn't matter. Then access to healthcare and prescriptions and pain management isn't important. If suffering is good, then what does it matter if it is just the result of illness and disability itself or also caused by poverty and hardship?

What's more, it cultivates an expectation that people with illnesses and disabilities must conform to a narrative of holiness. They cannot writhe or snivel in pain and desperation, they must become the wise blind guru, or the cheerful wheelchair-bound inspiration. They must keep their chins uplifted and teach us important lessons about human perseverance.

Those of us who are ill or disabled lose our humanity to these ideals. When we refuse to conform to this image of ecstatic suffering, we are shamed. If we speak out about the barriers we face, we are being too negative. If we admit to being unhappy, or even angry, at our lot, we are told by people who have never experienced the same level of pain to "think positive" or "look on the bright side." Our suffering is not something we feel, but something meant to inspire others.

When we abandon religion, we are even greater traitors than those who do so while happy or healthy. A comfortable person might be expected to forget religion, becoming complacent, only to return to God when times get hard. When people for whom times are always hard abandon religion, it challenges a foundational faith narrative. Suffering is supposed to bring us closer to God, to give us understanding of what he went through, to make us humble. We are supposed to be grateful for this lesson and act as an example to all those who forget faith when times are good. It is never considered how faith itself may have contributed to our suffering.

New Age and All Natural

Problems don't arise only from organized religions. In a society where the fad is to call oneself spiritual but not religious, disorganized and unorganized religions can be more prevalent. Their lack of organization aside, they lend themselves to just as many problems when they intersect with disability. Included among these are nonspiritual communities organized around a similar idea like a diet or lifestyle choice, such as all-natural movements.

Among the biggest problem created by these organizations, though not applicable to all nonorganized religions and cults, is the propagation of pseudoscience.

For example, a lot of Jenny McCarthy's antivax statements are linked to communities of autism parents who share a variety of nonscientific treatments for their children's condition. Some of these treatments can be relatively benign, but many of them are actively dangerous and abusive. Among these treatments are psychological therapies that are condemned as being damaging in the long term; pseudoscientific trust is also placed in homeopathy and alternative medicine that are at best useless and at worst actively harmful. As just one example, consider bleach enemas. While I am not saying that Jenny McCarthy engages in any of the listed abusive treatments, she has admitted to using hyperbaric chambers, and her antivax sentiments are already damaging enough.

These communities often spread hate and fear of autism rather than tolerance and acceptance. They are condemned by many autistic adults and other disability activists for encouraging abuse, and at times outright murder, of their children.

Other examples are proponents of the all-natural trend, who spread fear of "chemicals." These organizations might target genetically modified foods, prescription medications, processed foods, nonorganic produce, and so forth. They rely on the assumption that there is something significantly better about something natural vs unnatural. Of course, the definition of what constitutes natural is not applied consistently. For example, although living in a heated house could be seen as unnatural, there are very few sects that openly advocate in favor of homelessness.

They use fear of the unknown to prey on a scientifically ignorant populace. They warn of chemicals in food, for example, completely ignoring that even pure spring water is a chemical. That everything we ingest is a chemical. "Chemical" to them means anything that they believe to be fabricated in a laboratory. They assume that anything that is and was created in a lab cannot be found in nature.

Their efforts result in a social fear surrounding unnatural things like medications, medical treatments, psychological treatments, and so forth.

51 Worth Less

I've witnessed firsthand how the fight for women's rights often intersects with disability activism. Take abortion rights and access to birth control. I am under consideration for inclusion in various drug trials related to my disabilities. My participation would require that I not become pregnant. In order to ensure this, I would need access to birth control. This means that doctors or pharmacists who choose not to make birth control readily available don't just take away my rights as a person to make my own medical decisions, but they also actively put my health at risk. Even with my current medication, in the event that I got pregnant, having safe and easy access to abortion services would be necessary. As long as I am not in remission, being pregnant is thus a serious risk to my survival.

Similarly, my atheism and skepticism is brought into sharp focus by my struggles with medical conditions. Responding to religious and antiscience pundits is a daily act for those of us who are disabled. We face woo constantly, with it directed at us from friends, family members, and authority figures. Secular services are beneficial for more than just those who are nonreligious. Not every religious group or community has the same level of resources available, especially people belonging to smaller denominations, nontraditional or unorganized faiths, or faiths that fall outside the Judeo-Christian umbrella. By removing the integration of religion into a service, it makes the service available to more people regardless of their faith.

Disability activism highlights the importance of intersectionality since it can be the result as well as the cause of discrimination and marginalization. Many people who fall within the category of being trans, queer, women, people of color, and so forth live with the very real risk of physical harm and abuse, and as a result are at risk for anxiety, PTSD, depression, and physical impairment resulting from violence.

If we define disability as a physical or mental barrier from successfully and/or comfortably navigating our society, then race, gender, sexual, and gender orientation can all be seen as being disabilities. Perhaps disability activism should thus be seen as changing the world in such a way as to make the whole world more accessible to people of all genders, orientations, races, religions (or lack thereof), and physical and mental ability. Where potentially other social justice concerns differ from disability is that in the case of the former, the barriers are almost universally external, whereas in the case of the latter there do exist internal barriers as well, which may be further strengthened by the external.

Our society has such a negative attitude toward disability, however, that even people that fall into the socially accepted definition of that category struggle against being labeled as such. "I'm sick, but I'm not . . . you know . . . *disabled.*" It is hard to make the argument that disability is in any way a positive. Disability is painful, whether mental or physical. It makes your life harder. It can make it difficult to live a life that is socially deemed as worthwhile or productive. The personal aspects of disability won't change, but what can change are the external barriers that exist in our societies. By changing our concept of normalcy from "white cis straight able-bodied male who is financially secure" we can begin to change how our society handles differences.

Take mobility impairment for example. Most of our architecture and infrastructure is predicated on the assumption that people can walk. As a result, most buildings, sidewalks, and so forth are difficult to navigate for those of us for whom mobility is an issue. Where mobility disability is taken into account, it is usually in such a way as to be out of the way. Elevators are the most common solution, but of course elevators break down, are not consistently implemented, and, in the event of an emergency such as fire, are inaccessible. Imagine if we had a paradigm shift and instead based our architecture on the idea that a percentage of the population is not mobile? What if we replaced all stairwells with ramps? True, ramps take up more space then stairwells as they have to have lower incline then staircases do, but such a change would not negatively impact anyone. In fact, it would be beneficial to more than just the wheelchair bound. Parents with strollers, for example, would have a much easier time navigating, as would anyone who relies on wheel-based carriers. There would be a lower incidence of injury as falling down a ramp is less physically intense then falling down stairs.

Our culture's obsession with ranking relative value and worthiness is at the heart of many instances of oppression; white is more valuable than not-white, male is more valuable than female, cis is more valuable than trans, and so on and so forth. We do this with every aspect of our culture: someone who becomes a janitor or a blue-collar worker is seen as less valuable than someone who majors in business. In fact, blue-collar or no-collar work is seen as the domain of "stupid" people, and anyone who is "stupid" is inherently less valuable.

People with disabilities struggle with the concept of worthiness, or more specifically worthlessness, in particular. Our culture values productivity above many other things and the definitions of productivity can be limiting. When you exist in a body that forces you to spend entire days in bed for no other reason than because the pain you feel makes it too exhausting to get up, it can be difficult to feel like you have worth. When you see your friends and family members have to rearrange their lives around you, you get caught thinking over and over again, is it worth it? You feel like a burden. You feel worthless since by conventional standards you are not a productive member of society.

By the standards of our current society, we are worthless, and we are introduced to this idea every day. We hear about how people who rely on disability support payments are lazy. Every time someone talks about how they were "useless" because they spent the day in bed or at home is like a hot needle of shame shoved in our hearts. It is a reminder that as far as the majority of society is concerned, we are worthless.

Casual ableism is so prevalent in our society that in many ways what many would consider the most benign of insults are actually terms often used to marginalize people with disabilities. That's so lame, dumb, stupid, idiotic, retarded; he's so blind, slow, crazy, such a spaz—all these phrases have lost in the social memory the association with disability. And yet, that association exists. Imagine being a nonverbal child who knows that the designation for their impairment is used as a synonym for lacking in intelligence? Why is the opposite of cool or awesome a word that means having mobility impairment?

This casual ableism is prevalent in many social justice communities as well. Often, little to no thought is given on how a given subject, action, or word choice affects the disabled. Marches are organized without thought on how this limits participation by those who have difficulty walking. Having sign-language interpreters is the exception and not the rule. The activist behaviors most accessible to people with disabilities, such as the creation of online petitions, writing, posting on Facebook, is given the dubious label of slacktivism. This term is given without consideration of how, for some, these may be the only outlets for social change available to them. Many in the community see nothing wrong with comparing religious belief to mental illness.

Within the feminist community, when calling out the gas-lighting behavior that associates the word crazy with women, little-to-no thought is given to the inherent trouble with using crazy as a pejorative. What about women with bipolar disorder, depression, anxiety, PTSD? Is it okay to call them crazy since in some ways they are? Is it okay in that case to disregard what they have to say as unimportant, lacking in reason or merit?

When these concerns are brought up the thoughts are often dismissed as unimportant or at best thought exercises. When prominent atheist activists like Miri Mogilevsky of Brute Reason bring up the negative impact on atheists with mental disabilities caused by comparing religion to mental illness, the matter sparks some debate, but no pressure yet exists to enforce a change of behavior. The culprits had no fear of continuing their actions, even where they had previously done so to accommodate other social justice concerns.

In other cases where concerns over ableism or inaccessibility have been brought up, they are met with hostility and immediate dismissal.

When members of the community are dismissed or forced out from their positions due to their illness, we do not see the same level of public outcry as if someone were let go for reporting harassment, or forced out due to their race, beliefs, or gender expression. The marginalization or discrimination against people with disabilities doesn't cause scandals. It is at most a blip on the radar evoking the half-hearted response of "that sucks."

Disability concerns are an afterthought at most, if that. When it comes to activism, disability doesn't have the sex appeal of issues such as sexual orientation, gender, and race. When you are someone who struggles with disability and particularly with raising awareness of the issues as they exist within our communities, this dismissal creates a feeling of resentment. This is particularly the case when an inability to raise awareness on such issues means a continuation of the devastating impacts of living with these disabilities.

When a known member of the community struggled with potential homelessness as a result of their disability and inability to get the support they needed, the response was half-hearted at best, despite the money being asked for being less than outrageous. Raising it took a long time, putting pressure on the person in question as homelessness loomed. This occurred around the same time that the response to an unknown preacher losing his job due to a publicity stunt involving atheism led to tens of thousands of dollars being raised in a matter of days.

We as a community need to respond to the call to arms to support our own members—members whose everyday struggles are a lived manifestation of the need for atheist and feminist activism; members whose struggles are intimately intertwined with the professed concerns of this social movement. It is time to examine our own ableism. It is time to let wounded voices have a chance to speak. It is time to show the morality we claim of ourselves. A response to arms means more than just bringing awareness to a necessary social issue; it can quite literally save lives. I call on all those who call themselves humanists or intersectionalists to shut up and listen.

Part 4: Medical Marijuana

52 Herbal Medicine

I used to be terrified of cannabis. When I was in high school, I was chosen to be our school's representative at the regional antidrug advocacy seminar. I was terrified of drugs. I was convinced that if I ever tried even a single puff, that I would spiral into the depths of addiction and end up on the streets looking for another fix. This is what we were taught through the antidrug commercials, the talks at school, and so forth.

When I left the sheltered community I lived in for university, the reality seemed quite different than what I was taught. I saw responsible and intelligent individuals indulging from time to time without any negative consequence. The more I heard about marijuana from people how had used in the past, the more I came across studies, and the more I witnessed, the more I realized that what I had been taught was wrong. Marijuana wasn't some scary devil's weed. Although intellectually I knew that what I had been taught was wrong, I still feared touching the stuff. It just wasn't my thing. And that's perfectly okay.

I remember the first time I tried it. I was twenty-five years old, and I had been flaring for weeks. Every trip to the bathroom ended with me in tears. I felt like I had a rusty knitting needle sticking through my colon. I hadn't really eaten in several days, terrified of the pain it brought. My roommate at the time was a stoner. Strangely, knowing her made me a bit more afraid of marijuana rather than less. She had told me more than once that her cousin with Crohn's used it to help her with the pain. By this point I was desperate but still worried. I was allergic to smoke! Would it really work? Was I just setting myself up for some tragic result?

So I did what I usually do when questions such as this come up, I went to the Google. I browsed several scholarly sites, and what I found reassured me. A lot of studies out of the Netherlands showed a link between marijuana use and pain reduction in Crohn's patients. There was another site that showed the arguments for and against. The argument against boiled down to "it probably works but we don't know because we haven't studied it enough."

I decided to brave it.

To understand how I felt once I did, you would have to have been through extreme pain that lasted a long time, only to have it suddenly disappear. You would have to have been hungry and unable to eat, only to suddenly be able to enjoy food again. It was like having a sudden vacation in the midst of all this pain.

It was several months before I tried it again. Despite having experienced the benefits first hand, I was still at the mercy of internalized ableism and drug shaming. I didn't want to become one of *those* people.

It is hard to explain what it is like to experience pain every single day. Energy becomes a precious resource, like water in the desert, and like water it is rare and needs to be guarded carefully.

There is a lot of misinformation surrounding medical marijuana. On the one hand you have peddlers of misinformation making it out that marijuana is the very worst of drugs, creating rumors about how stoned people commit acts of violence. On the other hand you have the people elevating it to the status of panacea.

Cannabis works very well on a variety of symptoms. It is known for its pain control abilities. However, it can also help with nausea and relaxation. Different strains can also help with other symptoms, including anxiety, depression, and even certain types of focus problems. There are a variety of different conditions that benefit from different effects.

In my case I use it to control the chronic pain and nausea associated with Crohn's. It helps stimulate my appetite on the days when I am having a hard time eating. It helps my muscles relax, which in turn reduces arthritis pain. I have had prescription painkillers and anti-emetics, but when my Crohn's is flaring I have a hard time digesting pills. Oral medications don't work for me. They either don't work at all, or wear off long before I can take my next dose. A lot of painkillers also cause elevated nausea.

Marijuana on the other hand provides pain relief without involving my digestive system, without provoking nausea, and leaving me a lot more clearheaded than painkillers do.

But is the pain really that bad? Pain is natural! You don't look in pain.

Pain may be natural, but that doesn't make it good. Pain and inflammation have more long-term side effects than marijuana. Pain and inflammation can cause memory loss and reduced cognitive function, it can cause permanent nervous system changes. It can cause depression, change brain chemistry, supress appetite and sleep. It is a serious condition that a lot of people underestimate.

Chronic pain is not like the pain you get from a paper cut, or even a broken leg. It drains your energy your motivation.

When you live with chronic pain, you learn how not to show it. Pain becomes our reality so we have to learn to live our lives around it. I've laughed and danced around while my insides felt they were tearing. It costs me something to pretend not to be in pain, but the alternative is to never be able to have fun or to too often make other people uncomfortable.

A couple years ago I had my wisdom teeth removed. Before the operation I was hooked up to a machine that measured my heart rate, blood pressure, and oxygen saturation. I was talking happily with the nurses, and periodically, my heart rate would jump up for some time. The nurses kept trying to figure out what was going on, until finally one of them thought to ask me if I was having any pain, and I admitted I was. If not for the heart monitor, they would never have known. If trained professionals cannot tell when I am in pain, what hope do you have?

Okay, so why doesn't everyone do pot?

Pot is not a panacea. While it is very good for a variety of conditions, pot is also contraindicated for others, and not everyone reacts the same way. For example some people have had great luck with pot for migraines, while others find that marijuana makes their migraines worse.

While some people find it useful to help control anxiety, others find that the paranoia exacerbates it.

Even in my own use, I have learned that it doesn't work for all types of pain. It is great when dealing with the pain from my Crohn's and arthritis, but I have found that it doesn't work at all for pancreatitis and tooth-related pain.

Some people have adverse reactions to marijuana.

53 Are You Afraid of Getting Addicted?

Whenever I bring up the topic of medical marijuana, whether openly asking people to bring up myths and questions, or discussing it with someone who knows about my own use, the first topic to come up is invariably the one of addiction. People are concerned about the addictive properties, and like anytime a patient takes treatment for pain, there are the inevitable questions about whether we are worried about becoming addicted.

A lot of stoners will immediately start talking at this point about how marijuana is not addictive. There are conflicting studies on the matter, however. What is known is that marijuana is safe. With the conflictive information about addiction, it can be difficult to know what's what.

There are numerous studies that suggest that marijuana is not chemically addictive. So why the confusion?

The confusion comes from the matter of tolerance. One of the markers of addiction is building a tolerance to a medication and requiring a higher dose to achieve the same effect. Consistent (read: daily) use of marijuana can lead to an increased tolerance over time, which can lead to greater use. This would suggest that it is addictive.

However, if you talk to chronic users, whether medical or otherwise, they will tell you that all it takes to reset the tolerance is to skip a day here and there. While marijuana can stay in your system for several weeks, it leaves your system without significant withdrawal symptoms.

One of the myths surrounding addiction is the dichotomy between so-called chemical addiction and psychological addiction. To begin with, all addictions are psychological. They may feature a chemical dependency, but that is not always the case.

A chemical dependency on its own does not constitute addiction. If it did, a diabetic requiring insulin could be considered to be addicted to insulin. Similarly, patients who take certain medications, like prednisone, will develop a physical tolerance to medications, as their bodies start using the presence of a certain amount of the drug as a normal baseline, requiring more to yield the same therapeutic effect. In some cases, this will manifest as a series of negative side effects when the medication is not taken regularly, rather than as a need for higher doses.

Chemical dependency, however, can encourage the psychological component of addiction by adding a negative stimulus, such as in the case of people who experience severe withdrawal symptoms. In addition to the shot of dopamine created by the brain when the stimulus is ingested, the patient might have to deal with severe negative consequences for not interacting with the stimulus. Chemical dependency and the resulting physical tolerance can also make addiction more dangerous, as it increases the doses necessary to achieve the same reaction. This is when overdosing becomes a serious risk.

So if addiction is not a chemical dependency on its own, what is it?

Addiction is the *compulsive* engaging in either action or consumables that yields a positive stimulus, in which the continued engagements cause *distress* by interfering with life responsibilities or otherwise adversely affecting well-being.

But what does that mean? This is actually an extremely difficult question in and of itself, and in the field of psychology, one that frequently causes problems. The reason for this has to do with the nature of distress and the nature of compulsion.

54 It's My Fetish

To better explain what I mean by distress, I want to approach the idea from a different direction. I want to use a different psychological consideration: paraphilia. A very simplistic definition of paraphilia would be to call it fetishism. One example is cross-dressing (which is not the same thing as being transgender, to be perfectly clear).

One of the conversations that took place around the publication of the 5th edition of the Diagnostic and Statistical Manual of Mental Disorders was whether to include paraphilia. The cause for the debate has to do in part with the same discussion taking place here: understanding the psychological component of "distress" in determining whether something is a problem.

Let's take cross-dressing as an example. Imagine Ted. Ted likes to cross-dress in the privacy of his own home. He likes the way hose and silk feel, and he likes the little thrill of the forbidden he gets when he wears it. His wife knows and is okay with it. He has a good job, where he is never late, and has been a good steady employee for fifteen years. Clearly his cross-dressing isn't a problem, and is not causing distress. His emotional well-being is good. Everything is great.

Except one day, he is home alone engaging in his little fetish in the privacy of his own home. He doesn't realize that his curtain is flapping a little in the wind just as his boss happens to be walking down the street. The boss peeks in and sees Ted in his outfit.

The boss has a problem with cross-dressing. He thinks it is disgusting and that anyone who engages in it is a bad person. Now that he knows about Ted, he can't stand him. He fires him within the month on some trumped-up charge. Stressed by the lack of work, Ted has a fight with his wife who leaves him. Because he is out of work, he can't afford to see friends as often as he would like to. The cross-dressing has now created distress, so is it a problem?

On the one hand we have a clear link between Ted's cross-dressing and his distress. On the other hand, the distress is not the result of him seeking a certain stimulus regardless of consequences, but is the result of someone else's problem with what he does. So is the cross-dressing to blame, or is the person who holds bigoted opinions the one who has a problem?

So how does this relate to addiction? In determining whether someone has a problem with an action or substance, it can be difficult to isolate the root impetus behind the distress.

Take my own pot use for example. Due to my disability, I am unable to work. This is in part due to my need for frequent pain treatment, though this is by no means the only or even the most pressing reason why I am unable to work. In fact, even if my pain treatments were 100 percent not an issue, I would still be far from able to work.

Pot use, even when legal, exposes people to a large amount of shaming. This can put medical users like me in a position where we are forced to choose between being able to medicate and going out in public. Since often the symptoms can be debilitating in and of themselves, it could mean that the choice is not much of one either way.

So in my case we have an instance in which distress is caused: my social life is limited and I struggle financially. On the surface this might suggest that the medical marijuana is a problem. However, in truth the root cause of both of these circumstances is not my pot use but rather my disability to begin with. The perception becomes one of a person taking advantage of so-called free money to sit around and get high. What this ignores is the severity of circumstance that put me in that position.

The existence of symptoms creating a need for treatment means that the impetus behind seeking a certain stimulus can be nearly impossible to determine. Is it addiction, or is it a need to be able to eat dinner for the first time in three days? Is it addiction, or is it trying to make some of your pain go away? Determining the truth can be nearly impossible from the outside, since there is a strong motivation to use either way.

Some people might point to the fact that some medical marijuana patients are not able to use legally. As a result they are risking jail time in order to continue using. Clearly this must be an indication of a problem such as addiction, right? Wrong. Once again, the nature of disability and pain gets in the way. The person in question might not be seeking marijuana because they feel the drive to consume it regardless of the consequences, but because the alternative is experiencing severe symptoms. It might be that the symptoms of the disease themselves are worse than the risk of jail time. In many cases, the choice is not simply whether to risk jail or risk a bit of pain. Rather, the choice might actually be to risk jail or risk torturous pain—or even death. To put it another way: would you consider a diabetic an addict if insulin were illegal?

55 So What?

In answer to the question of whether marijuana can be addictive, the answer is yes. Marijuana can be addictive. While it can foster some physical tolerance, it does not really create a chemical dependency, which is why many will insist that it isn't.

That is not enough of a reason to make it illegal. Caffeine, sex, sugar, shopping, gambling, anything that causes your brain to produce dopamine can become addictive. The reason our society has this perception that addictive things must be made illegal is because of a study several years ago, featuring rats isolated in cages, which suggested that availability was all that was needed to encourage addiction.

This study formulated our entire social opinion of addiction. It was used to instigate extreme laws banning a series of narcotic substances in order to prevent addiction. Any slight attention to drug statistics of the last several years will confirm that those laws were an absolute failure. The draconian drug laws have actually led to higher levels of addiction rather than lower.

The study failed to take into account that rats are social creatures. If applied to humans, it would be the equivalent of giving drugs to inmates in solitary confinement. The psychological impact of this was not taken into account. A second series of studies looked at rats that were kept in a more pleasing community environment. Although the study was shut down before enough data could be collected, the gathered results showed evidence that in a positive psychological environment, simple availability is not enough to foster or maintain addiction.

While not enough information has been gathered as of yet to make a definitive conclusion, results from countries that have implemented more progressive drug policies suggest that legalization is significantly more effective in eliminating addiction than punitive measures. This is in part because legalization reduces the likelihood that an addiction would mean complete social isolation and an inability to seek treatment.

This suggests that the biggest risk factors for addiction are different forms of isolation. So shaming disabled medical marijuana users, and thus isolating them even further, increases the possibility for addiction to occur. Isolating drug addicts, in the form of imprisonment, can make the hold of addiction stronger.

So how do we prevent addiction in disabled patients taking potentially addictive medications?

By reducing the causes of isolation imposed on those of us who have them. These causes include poverty, social stigma and shaming of medication use, ableism, and so forth. And it doesn't stop there. In order to truly protect people from addiction, we would have to address racism, sexism, transantagonism, and all of the other oppressions intersecting within the broader concept of kyriarchy. That's a tall order, but not half as costly as the damage done by our society's deep misunderstanding of chronic illness and "addiction."

56 So Are You Afraid of Getting Addicted?

Yes. It would be a lie to say that I have never worried about the possibility of getting addicted to pot, or any other pain medication I've taken for that matter. I wonder about it every time I stay home so that I can smoke. I think about it every time I have to medicate before noon. I think about it every time someone brings it up.

Social shaming regarding taking pain medication, regardless of what kind, has made sure that most people with chronic pain feel guilty for medicating. Sometimes this fear goes so far as to stop us from medicating even when we should. We ignore more pain than is safe, because we want to make sure that no one thinks that we might be addicted. We are afraid of getting labelled an addict because that label will mean the end of consistent treatment and the loss of whatever trust doctors had in our veracity.

What scares me more, though, are the long-term results of pain. I am afraid of the depression that I slip into when my body hurts so much that killing myself seems like a logical solution to make the pain stop. I am afraid of watching myself waste away again. I am afraid of needing to have my bowels removed and needing surgery after countless surgery because my body won't stop attacking itself. In other words, like many people who use medicine to treat their conditions, I am more afraid of my illness than I am of some potential risk of becoming addicted.

57 What's Stopping Use?

In many places, medical marijuana is still not legal, but even in places where it is, like Canada, challenges to getting the drug remain. While my experience is limited to Canada, one of the first and biggest barriers to medical marijuana is a lack of information as to how to go about getting a prescription. It used to be that you had to fill out a large complicated set of forms to be submitted to Health Canada. The application would then be handled by some bureaucratic process at which point you would be approved or denied.

In March 2014 the rules changed. Now, instead of filling out a Health Canada form, you fill out a form directly with your choice of dispensary. The Health Canada website provides you with a list of licensed dispensaries, and most of them have their forms available online.

The forms include two parts: personal information and doctor prescription. The prescription form has to be filled out by a medical doctor, and includes dosage information as well as the doctor's office information.

The forms are mailed to the dispensary, which confirms that the doctor who filled out the prescription is properly licensed, and you become a registered patient.

While many patients are uninformed, so too are doctors. When I first wanted a prescription, I asked my GI for it. He said no. I was surprised since he actually seemed supportive of my occasional use.

Over the next few months, whenever marijuana came up with other doctors, like those at the ER, they recommended that I get a prescription. I was torn. Doctors seemed supportive of the general idea, yet I couldn't manage to get a prescription. Finally, I decided to bring it up with my GI again and asked why he was unwilling to give me one.

It turned out that my doctor was under the impression that a condition had to be fatal in order to allow for the use of medical marijuana. Even though he thought that pot would be beneficial for me, he believed he wasn't allowed to prescribe it for me.

Other doctors are unaware of the current available research. I had one ER doctor believe that marijuana was contraindicated for Crohn's even though Crohn's is one of the few conditions that have had studies confirming the benefit of marijuana.

Patients are not the only people being fed misinformation about medical marijuana. Doctors are just as likely to have mistaken ideas about its use, its addictive properties, and so forth. The new rule changes make doctors the gatekeepers to prescriptions, but no efforts have been made to properly educate them. This leaves it up to patients to educate them or find a sympathetic doctor.

Even those patients who are more knowledgeable in the effects and use of marijuana may find it difficult to find a sympathetic doctor. It is counterintuitive to most patients to push their doctors for explanations. Since there is the fear of being labeled a drug seeker, patients might also worry about seeming overeager about the acquisition of a prescription.

As per the new rules, you have to register with a dispensary. While it appears that Health Canada allows you to register with two at once, most dispensaries themselves insist on being your only provider. As a result, patients are dependent on the strains available at one dispensary. This limits a patient's ability to find the strains that work best for them.

If the dispensary runs out of the strains that work, the patient might find themselves without their meds for however long it takes for a new working strain to be available.

Other places where marijuana is legal work with a prescription system where you have a card and can bring it to different dispensaries.

58 Legalize It

In many places in North America, as well as the rest of the world, marijuana is still illegal. Medical users are sometimes forced to go to dealers to meet their needs. This is true whether someone is on chemotherapy looking for relief, or has some other medical reason.

For some people, medical marijuana is one of the only things that helps with their condition. It can be a matter of desperation if a lack of access means living in constant pain. For the people who use it to control mental-health conditions, the need to have access to your medication can be even more essential. Imagine for example those who use the uplifting effects to control their suicidal tendencies?

Although nominally legal in certain U.S. states, federal agents have raided "legal" grow-ops in the past, since marijuana continues to be illegal on the federal level. This creates an especially difficult situation for people who have reason to be particularly careful about adherence to federal laws, even when they contradict state law. This includes those who are in the midst of a citizenship application or work for the federal government.

Questionable legality may also create problems at workplaces that do drug testing.

Another barrier is portability. Since the legality of marijuana is different from place to place, you might not be able to have access to your medication when you travel. This can make things like visiting family difficult. Within the United States, legality can change from state to state. While in Canada it is federally approved across the provinces, those with reason to travel to the United States are not allowed to cross the border with their medication.

This may seem reasonable at first because of medical marijuana's questionable legal status, but consider that this is not true of any other medication. At need one can arrange to bring any other prescription with them and even have it filled if needed at pharmacies in the United States.

Similarly, it can be difficult to know where it is safe to take your meds. Pain and symptoms strike anywhere. For example, if you experience pain due to eating, eating out might be difficult. If you are visiting friends you might be unable to take your pain medication with you. Smoking in public is awkward. If people think you are smoking tobacco you run the risk of being verbally assaulted for your choice. If they realize you are smoking pot, you run the risk of having the police called on you, being yelled at, being threatened, and so forth.

What's more, the rules regulating where a patient is allowed to smoke are unclear. On the one hand, a patient should be able to medicate within reason, anywhere that they are able to go. Due to the air-contaminating nature of smoking marijuana, at the very least medical marijuana patients should be able to medicate wherever cigarettes are allowed.

Despite this being the case, there is some suggestion that a prescription applies only to private residences. This in turn means that those without a place of their own may not have a place to legally medicate at all if their family or friends do not allow it in their homes. This adds an additional constraint on people trying to decide whether they should go out and suffer through pain or stay in and medicate.

59 Stoner Guilt

The biggest repellent to medical marijuana use is not bureaucracy or the law, however. It is shaming. This comes in many varieties, but it is consistently listed as the biggest barrier experienced by medical users. There are the "concerned-and-caring" shamers, the fear-mongers, the naturalists, the religiously motivated, and so on. The people who engage in this behavior may fall into various categories even in one conversation.

Medical marijuana users, whether they have a prescription or not, are made to feel ashamed. We are portrayed in media as being slow-witted, while conservative news paints us as being violent criminals. Many of us have to contend with disapproving relatives who condescendingly explain to us everything that is wrong with us for deciding to treat our pain. Or who use misinformation to try and convince us that what we are doing is wrong, even in the face of overwhelming evidence to the contrary.

Medical marijuana users are often accused of faking the severity of our pain. In other instances, we are expected to perform pain to justify its use. We will have people questioning us, and questioning whether we are *really* in pain. Or whether the pain is really bad enough to require such *drastic* measures.

Even among less-scientifically-illiterate religions that encourage proper medical care, the use of medical marijuana is characterized as a sin. Those users in more conservative religions risk being shunned.

Of course, often when people are questioned about their objections to marijuana, you discover that their disagreement seems to be about painkillers in general. Just the act of treating pain is seen as an act of weakness, instead of the necessity it really is.

As a result, patients can find it difficult to take their medication. Those who live in apartments have to be careful to not let the distinctive smell bother their neighbors. They run the risk of having disapproving landlords pointlessly hassle them or even threaten eviction.

Staying with family can create a need to hide your use, or create awkward situations when you have to medicate. Patients can find themselves being cornered and lectured while they are medicating or shortly afterward. They might be forbidden from taking the medication on the property and be forced to go elsewhere if they need to address their symptoms because of this ongoing lack of acceptance of marijuana as medication rather than recreation.

In deference to their parents' or friends' discomfort, some patients are able to go a certain time without their medication. This is especially true if their use is already sparing, or if they have access to other medications that can help treat their symptoms. Other patients, myself among them, might have medical marijuana as the only prescription for their symptoms, and thus being separated from this medication for a significant period of time means greater hardship.

60 It's Expensize

Since it is a relatively new drug from the standpoint of Western medicine, many insurance companies don't cover prescription marijuana as of yet. Even the provincial coverage available to those on government benefits does not cover medical marijuana. Many of the people relying on medical marijuana are people who have fairly severe disabilities. Many are struggling financially as a result of their illness, so the added financial burden of having to pay for this uncovered prescription can be particularly difficult.

For example, I am on ODSP, which provides me with some prescription coverage, but marijuana is not covered s of this writing. The cost at my dispensary averages about $10 per gram, and the standard prescriptions is one gram per day. This means that for a full month's prescription I have to find $300. Most months I've been able to average significantly less than that, but some months are more difficult than others. Because the majority of my money comes from disability, I have to budget very carefully. After covering my monthly bills, there isn't always a lot of money left behind to cover groceries and other expenses, so even cutting my prescription in half represents quite a big chunk of the money I have.

What makes it more difficult is when dispensaries have a minimum order, some as much as $100. Being forced to go without pain medication can mean more than more pain. It can cost you money as well if you find yourself eating out more because pain is draining you of energy. It can mean a trip to the hospital and even an admission.

Ultimately all of the barriers come from the same source: misinformation piled on an underlying social culture of ableism.

Part 5: A Little Friendly Advice

61 What Not to Do, or How Not to Help

After sharing all my experiences with disability, I want to take a moment to offer some advice on how *not* to interact with people with disabilities. This list is generated from my experience, and so it might not be completely comprehensive and applicable to all disabled people. That said, I think it provides some insight into how to be a supportive ally to those of us with disabilities.

Don't Police My Health. At times, friends have been a little *too* understanding of the limitations my disabilities cause me, and have become too concerned about everything I do. This can quickly cross the line from concern into policing behavior. While I appreciate that the friend is worried about me, asking me constantly whether I should be eating or drinking something, or whether I should be engaging in some activity, ultimately implies that they know more about my health than I do.

It gets particularly bad when I am doing something that really isn't best for my health, be it drinking alcohol or coffee, indulging in a dairy product or some treat that I never allow myself to eat, or lifting a box that is too heavy for me. We all indulge in unhealthy behaviors from time to time. Yes, my conditions might have more intense consequences than those of most people, but trust me to assess my own risk tolerance in what I can handle.

Don't Compare Me to Other People with Chronic Illnesses or Disabilities, Even If They Have the Same One(s). I get this one a lot: "My mom has Crohn's and it never bothered *her* this much" or "Well, my doctor has Crohn's and she totally managed to make a career and is well off, so why can't you do the same?" The assumption here is that the person they are talking to is somehow exaggerating or lying about how they are handling their disorder.

It is insulting, but it is also based on bad examples. Every case and every person is different. There are plenty of people out there with Crohn's, with arthritis, and with other disabilities, who have milder versions of these conditions. Their symptoms can be minor, or may have responded well to medication. They may have a higher pain tolerance, while another person may have other reasons why they cannot cope as well. In comparing different people with disabilities you are ultimately taking away their individuality and lumping everyone into the same pigeonhole.

Not only that, but not everyone is comfortable sharing the extent of their disability with everyone else. Your mom may have chosen to hide how much pain she was in so as not to worry you. Your doctor may have had a difficult set of years that she doesn't talk about. You cannot know how someone's illness affects them unless you live in their skin.

Don't Tell Me I Don't Look Sick. Tell me, how does chronically ill or disabled look? How do you see stomach distress, or depression, or pain? There may be ways that people act when they feel a certain way, but what if someone is used to it? If I feel pain every single day, am I still supposed to wince at every cramp? Illness and disability don't come with a mark of Cain that shows it to the world. If I don't always appear sick it's because my illness is not a performance for your benefit.

You may think you are being nice by telling me that I don't look like a sick person, but in reality, you are making it seem like you don't believe me. Given the difficulties I've faced—and continue to face—in trying to have my condition acknowledged, such compliments, well-meaning as they may be, only serve to frighten me.

Don't Ask Whether I Have Tried X, Y, or Z. You are likely not a doctor and, even if you are, you are not my doctor. Some article you read in *Not-a-Science-Journal* daily does not medical advice make. If it is a legitimate treatment, I have probably tried it already. If it isn't, I don't want to know about it. I simply do not have the energy to explain to a hundred different people why eating more salad is such a bad idea for me, or why starting a running regime is impossible.

What is worse is when people become convinced that their lifestyle choice is a magical cure all. I respect people who decide to go gluten-free, or vegan, or whatnot, but it is not going to cure my Crohn's. While marijuana manages my symptoms pretty well, it is not going to cure it. It is a drain on my energy to have to explain to every person the various idiosyncrasies of Crohn's.

Of course, there are exceptions. If I ask you for advice that is obviously a time to share what you think. Alternatively, if you suffer from the same disorder I do and want to share what worked, that is okay as well. Assuming, of course, that you are not being too pushy and maintain an understanding that what worked for you might not work for me.

Don't Send Me Articles You Have Read without Asking. So you've found an interesting article that deals with my condition and you just have to share it with me. This is in many ways better than simply telling me about it like in the above example, but the end result is often me being swamped with articles often saying the same thing. My best suggestion is that if you have found an article that you honestly think I would find interesting, ask me if it is okay to send it first. I might let you know that I've already read it, or I might point out a problem with the source, or I might be very thankful. But by giving me the choice you are making it clear that you don't want to pressure me into anything.

Don't Encourage Me to Just Think Positive. I hate this one so much. There are many variations of this, including "Pain is all in your head," "Just don't focus on the bad things," and so forth. It comes from the idea that all disability comes from the mind and that the only thing getting in my way is attitude. This one is in particular often aimed at those of us who suffer from depression, the idea being that depression is just a crisis of attitude, that we wouldn't be depressed anymore if we would just think more positively. This idea ignores scientific evidence and, worse yet, serves to silence anyone who points out the problems in how our society deals with the ill, the disabled, and the mentally ill. Positive thinking won't cure my condition; it won't make my pain go away.

While it is true that meditation and certain mental exercises can help lessen symptoms in some people, it is not a cure, nor will it work for everyone. Many people who struggle with illnesses already work hard to cultivate a positive attitude, but that won't suddenly make the negatives disappear. Moreover, talking about the negatives can help people feel better, but the fear of being told to think positive and not wallow in negativity may keep people from doing the very thing that can actually help them.

Don't Express Concern That I'm So Young. This one is obviously limited to those of us who still fall into the young category, however defined. It stems from the idea that bad things don't happen to young people. We are not supposed to suffer joint pain, or get sick in a way that puts our lives at risk, because that is too sad.

The "but you're so young" comment highlights our abnormality or, perhaps, makes us wonder if the speaker suspects that we may be lying. It also reminds us that this will be our life for a long time, that we can potentially expect to have to deal with this infirmary for forty, fifty, sixty years or more. It is also a harsh reminder that my conditions might actually shorten my overall lifespan. Can I really expect to live to a ripe old age when I have already been so near death in my twenties?

In my case, such comments are also a reminder that my conditions were allowed to severely affect my life for so long before they were taken seriously because of the mistaken concept that young people cannot be seriously ill. So much of my pain might have been avoided if doctors had looked at my symptoms rather than my age.

Don't Offer an Opinion about Whether I Should Ever Have Kids. Interestingly, I have only heard the "I guess that means you won't have kids" directed at women.

It is not usually phrased that way. Often it will follow some variation of "how does this affect your ability to have kids?" I have also had people express opinions that I shouldn't have kids because I might pass on my condition, or my body is too damaged to be able to carry a pregnancy, or that I may not be physically able to meet the needs of a small child. Some have even argued that it is irresponsible for someone who is sick to have kids. None of this comes from doctors, of course. Interestingly, male friends with disabilities don't seem to get asked this question. My decision about whether or not to have kids is deeply personal. Unless you are someone with whom I would be having these kids, or my doctor, your opinion about is completely irrelevant. I will make that decision myself.

I will do so in consultation with my doctor to find out what the risks are both to me and to my potential offspring.

Anyone planning to have a children must face the risk that their children may be sick. My parents don't have Crohn's, they don't have arthritis, and yet they had a child with both. The healthy and able-bodied lie to themselves if they believe that this risk assessment belongs only to those of us who are sick.

When you say you don't think I should have kids, even if it is because you worry about my ability to do so and survive, you are involving yourself in a very personal decision. You are making that decision harder for me because now I know that if I decide to have kids, I won't have your support—and if you are a friend, your support matters to me. You are also saying, though I know this is probably not your intent, that people with my condition can't make good parents.

Don't Compare Your Flu to My Condition. I get the impulse toward empathy and comparative experience to funnel understanding, but no, you don't know exactly what I am going through. At most, you are at a 1 percent understanding of what I am going through. Your flu might have similar symptoms to Crohn's, but it has a start and it has an end. Your body, when you get the flu, isn't already exhausted from having gone through those same symptoms for months or even years. You have an expectation that at some point the flu will end. Yes, the flu is terrible, but it is a completely different experience. By comparing them, you are minimizing my experience. Everyone gets the flu from time to time, not everyone gets Crohn's. When you have the flu, you don't get the same number of people determined to tell you why it is all your fault. When you have the flu, you can take the time you need to get better. When you have Crohn's you don't have that option because it won't get better. You have to continue trying to live your life.

Don't Think I Want to Just Stay Home All Day and Do Nothing. What exactly do people imagine I do all day? Do you think I am at home watching TV, reading, doing fun relaxing activities? I'm not. In most cases I am spending my morning trying to find the energy to get out of bed, because coming awake and getting up takes up more energy than I have. I am trying to ignore pain that makes me want to curl up and cry. The smell of food makes me nauseated even if I haven't eaten in hours, or days, and I know that I have to force myself to eat something. And then I have to hope that it will stay down.

I am not making the decision to stay home. Often I have no choice. I am completely isolated from friends, from family, because I don't have the energy to go out or to entertain. When you are stuck at home like that, you are trapped. You don't want to stay at home. You would love to go out, to do some shopping, to meet up with friends, see a movie, just get out of the house. But you can't. And you don't know when you will be able to. Because you just don't have the energy.

Don't Say You Think I'm *Still* Hot. *Oh thank you so much.* Your magic ability to see past my illness to the beauty that exists within me suddenly cures all the problems and anxieties that stem from society's perception of people with disabilities as being unattractive or desexualized.

I get that you think you are being nice, but telling me about how you think I am hot despite my disability is not just unhelpful but is actually a symptom of the problem. Why shouldn't you think that I am attractive? My disability doesn't stop me from being a person with sexual desires or sex appeal; it is our society that tells us that it should stop me. When you say that you "still" think I am hot, it implies that there is a reason you shouldn't. Even more than that, it is not helpful to me in the least that you think I am attractive. Unless you are someone I am looking to engage in a relationship with, then your personal opinion is irrelevant to me.

Don't Shame My Need for Medications. Taking medication isn't pleasant. Taking medication can be physically painful—like having to get an injection—or can cause side effects—like exhaustion, nausea, etc. It is not something that I enjoy. I don't take them because they are fun. When I was on subcutaneous injections, I had to talk myself into them, and this was despite knowing that they would bring relief, that they were doing me some good. I take my medications, because not taking them is a worse alternative. And then you come along and decide to make my life more difficult by shaming me and telling me all about how what I am doing is poisoning myself. I don't need to deal with your shaming about how I am overmedicated, or how I should be chasing "natural" alternatives instead.

Don't Use Ableist Language. Language plays an integral role in how people view things. Words that are used as slurs denote who we as a society see as lesser. It is thus not surprising that a series of words associated with one or more disabilities have become pejoratives in the English language. Words like retard are already becoming social unacceptable, though not as widely unacceptable as they should be. Other words that are ableist include idiot, stupid, lame, cretin, dumb, spaz/spastic, gimp, crazy, insane, and so forth.

If you want to be supportive of people with disabilities, stop contributing to a language culture that uses our existence as an insult.

Don't Guilt Me or Get Mad at Me for Having to Cancel Plans. I wish I could go to every event that I wanted to. Often, I will agree to go to something—an event, a party, a get-together—and then on the day of the event I wake up in pain, or sick, or just completely lacking in energy and I have to make the decision not to go. I hate cancelling plans because I don't want to disappoint you, but sometimes I have no choice. Going could mean spending the whole time in the bathroom, or being unresponsive, or it could mean that I spend the next week sick and in pain because I didn't treat my symptoms right away. I already feel bad about cancelling, and having you get mad at me or guilt me by reminding me of all the other times I cancelled isn't helpful. It makes me wary of agreeing to hang out with you in future, since I cannot guarantee I won't have to cancel again.

62 What to Do, or How to Help

Now that the "don'ts" are out of the way, I do get asked from time to time how people can be helpful to me and others with disabilities. Here are some suggestions.

Do Offer a Helping Hand, Not Just to Me but Also to My Significant Other. Being sick is draining. It can take a lot of effort to make dinner, to clean the house, or to take care of any assortment of errands that need to be done on a given day. What's more, a lot of times, my partner ends up having to handle the brunt of the work, from dishes to vacuuming, in addition to her own responsibilities like work and studies. Some of the most helpful things that friends have done is help with the cleanup when they come over. I have one friend who will sometimes do the dishes after a session of Dungeons and Dragons, saying she wanted to do it as thanks for the awesome meal we provided. If you really want to help out a friend with chronic pain or illness, doing little things to make their lives easier is a big deal. Bring over some extra food you made (but ask first about any dietary restrictions they may have), or offer to pick up some groceries for them since you are heading that way anyway. The offer won't always be accepted, but if made casually and without the air of condescension and charity, it will go a long way toward us knowing that we can rely on you if we really do need help.

Do Arrange for Low-Energy Hangouts. I hate having to cancel on parties or going out with friends. Being sick and disabled makes me feel so isolated. Even planning an evening in my own home can be too much energy since

I have to clean ahead of time, prepare food, entertain during the event, and clean up afterward. It becomes a catch-22 situation where I don't have enough energy to go out or entertain, but doing neither leaves me feeling depressed and drains my energy as well. If you want to help without taxing my energy, why not bring over a couple of movies or TV shows and some takeout. Take the burden off of me to provide entertainment and food.

Do Let Me Complain. This may seem strange, but sometimes all I want is to be able to rant about how things suck without someone trying to tell me to think positive, or trying to come up with solutions. I need to be able to get things off my chest and know that someone is listening. That can be very hard to find. Be that person. Let me have a moment from time to time to indulge in the catharsis of talking about how what is going on in my life is messed up, unfair, and sucks.

Do Check in from Time to Time. Whether you are struggling from physical illness or mental illness, it can be difficult to reach out to people. You don't want to overwhelm them with your problems. You don't want to be the downer. Sometimes, you just assume that people don't care. Checking in from time to time, asking them how they are doing, if they want to talk, or even just reminding them you are there, can be huge in reducing the social isolation they may be feeling. It can help push away the anxious thoughts that we are a burden on you, on society, and on everyone else.

Do Let Me Be There for You. Although it can be frustrating when people assume they know what we feel like when they deal with a flu or something along those lines, that doesn't mean that you have to hide from me that you are having a bad time. I have had people tell me that they didn't want to complain about their monetary problems or health problems with me because I have it so much worse and they felt guilty. I want to be there for you. I don't think your problems are less important just because they are different from mine. I have no less sympathy for you when you are struggling with a bad cold or a bad flu. I know they suck. And being able to help someone else—whether materially or just by being an ear for your complaints—can help me feel like I, too, have something to contribute. It helps me feel like I am not just a recipient but also a useful person in my own right as well.

When you don't let me be there for you, you end up isolating me. Rather than being your friend, I end up being a symbol of how things could be worse, and that's no fun.

Do Offer Hugs (but Ask before Touching). A lot of conditions can make touch painful. Even when it doesn't, anxiety and other such issues can make touch feel like an attack, or make one feel claustrophobic. I love hugs, but there are times when I cannot handle them, times when even the gentlest pressure can be too much. So ask first. But like many human beings, I am also comforted by physical contact. Sometimes a hug can make me feel better; it can make me feel connected to other people and lift my spirits. So offer hugs, but ask first. And if I have to refuse, please don't take it personally, but understand that at that moment a hug will create more pain than it will take away.

Do Be a Safe Space. One of the biggest problems when you struggle with physical and mental disability is that it can be difficult to know who to trust, with what, and when. I am scared of being a burden on people, of being a downer, or of being considered too demanding. Like a lot of people, I often let things slide or put myself in harm's way because it is easier than speaking up. If you spend hours making dinner that includes things I cannot eat, I don't want to be the ingrate who doesn't eat, but eating it might mean being incapacitated later in the evening. It gets to be exhausting having to remind people what I can and can't do, of having to remind them to slow down when we walk, or having to excuse myself from activities that might be too physically intense. Be my safe space. Be someone I don't have to worry about cancelling with, or explaining my limitations to. Be my support network, someone I can count on if things are rough and I ask for help.

Do Perform Your Own Research and Check Your Privilege. Having to explain to a bunch of different people over and over again what Crohn's is, what the difficulties of being disabled are, what ableism is, can get exhausting. Having to call you or others on ableism is also exhausting and risky for me. If you really want to be a big help to me, educate yourself. Find out what ableism is and how it influences our society. Read what I and other people have written about the realities of living with a disability.

Don't Expect Me to Have to Explain Every Little Thing for You. If I do take the risk to call you on something, don't waste the precious little energy I have telling me that your intentions were good. Intentions matter only insomuch as I might be more patient with you the first time or two. Ultimately, what matters is the harm your actions or speech may be causing. You might not have meant to bump into me, but that doesn't mean I don't have a right to get upset or expect an apology when I fall to the ground as a result. Same thing applies.

Try to remember that an apology tells me that you are listening and that you will try to do better next time. An explanation tells me that you are more concerned about the blow I struck against your pride than by the hurt you might have caused by your actions, inadvertent though they may have been.

Do Ask Me If It Is Okay to Ask Questions. I actually don't mind educating people about Crohn's. I have a pretty high comfort level for discussing personal details, as should be obvious by the very existence of this book, but this is not the case for everyone. In fact, this is not the case for most people. Telling you about my disability means letting you know things that may be intensely personal and potentially humiliating. Not everyone is comfortable making themselves so vulnerable.

Before asking me questions about my medical history, ask if it is okay to do so and respect my answer. Understand that it is not my job to educate you and I don't owe you any personal information. I also may have reasons why I don't want to discuss things at a particulat time. Perhaps the location is too public and I don't want to talk about certain issues there. Perhaps I have had a really bad time with my health lately and discussing it makes me more aware of the pain I am in. There are many reasons why I may not want to share information with you at any given moment and you must respect that. The moment you start feeling entitled to answers you need to stop.

Consider, also, that you may be contributing to my discomfort unnecessarily, as many questions can easily be answered through a little online research.

Do Let Me Control the Speed When Walking. It may seem like such a small thing, but the impact is huge. Often I struggle to keep up with other people. This is especially true when there is a big group walking somewhere together. Many times I have been put in a situation where I had to make the choice between causing myself pain by trying to keep up with people or getting left behind. Other times, I have to keep calling to people, letting them know they are walking too fast. When this happens over and over again, this makes walking anywhere too much of a chore for me, so I avoid it.

Trying to keep up is not only exhausting because it puts undue pressure on already damaged joints, but it is also isolating and unpleasant. Having to remind people constantly makes me feel guilty, so I end up trying to push myself more than I should—which means dealing with pain for the next few days. I understand that my pace is slow and that this can be frustrating, and I understand that it can be difficult to remember to walk at a pace that may be quite different from your natural speed, but if you actually care about my well-being and feelings, letting me set the pace goes a long way.

Do Ask. Ultimately, the best thing to do is ask me or anyone else what you can do to help. I will appreciate the offers. If you have specific ideas, like driving me to appointments, picking up my groceries, or helping me around the house, you can mention those. It helps give me an idea of what you are offering. By asking me how you can help me, or make me feel more welcomed, you let me know that suggestions are welcome and okay. If I say thank you but refuse help, accept that. I might not need help at that moment, or I might have other reasons for refusing.

Also, keep in mind the difference between "may I help you?" and "how may I help you?" Some people will nominally ask if they can help, and rather than waiting for an answer will proceed to do what they assume is help. This might mean grabbing the arm of a blind person, pushing a wheelchair, or any other assortment of actions. While the person thinks they are being helpful, they could be causing more harm than good. More importantly, however, they are not respecting bodily autonomy. I may not want you to touch me. I might experience pain from you doing so. I may suffer some other consequence. Ultimately, I have a right to say no and to set my own boundaries. Anyone who refuses to respect the boundaries of a person with a disability is treating us as less than human and is not an ally.

Everyone is different and what they need will differ. I know people who benefit from being able to look at their phones during social interaction since it lessens their anxiety. There are others who benefit from having someone watch their kids for a few hours so that they can get a bit of time for self-care. There is any number of little things that can go a long way toward creating a more comfortable environment for those of us struggling with disability.

63 What Can Atheist Groups Do

If religion is so bad on matters of disability, why do so many disabled people continue to have faith? Surely there should be an increase of people with disabilities joining atheist movements, such as there is among other persecuted minorities like homosexuals and trans folk. Yet, this appears not to be the case. Is it because people with disabilities are impaired cognitively? No. It is because for many of us, religion can be a source of aid.

Religious communities are often better organized to provide aid than secular ones. Since religion markets itself as a source of comfort, its primary targets are people who need comforting. Namely those who struggle. This is why struggling minorities, such as people in poverty, seniors, people of color, people with disabilities, and women are more often associated with a church than other such populations.

Churches can provide access to child care, financial assistance, clothing, food, and many other essentials—all for free, provided you are a member of the church. Religious organizations are also more likely to provide attendant home care and friendly visits by volunteers than secular ones. As a result, regardless of faith, religion becomes a lifeline for struggling people.

For those of us who were once a part of a religious community but who have since become atheists, the consequences stemming from our disability are direr than if we remained participants and congregants of our former religions.

This is not because religious people are inherently more moral. In fact, morality doesn't play into it at all. What religions have that the atheist movement still lacks is infrastructure and community—more specifically, an infrastructure-based community that understands that the best way to keep its numbers is to provide services that make it unappealing and at times impossible to leave. The services can be provided officially by religious institutions or unofficially by parishioners who organize themselves.

In the interest of improving the lives of disabled atheists I want to offer some examples of things that the atheist community as a whole can do to help those of us who struggle.

Offer Ride Programs. One of the biggest challenges faced by people with disabilities, regardless of their financial status, is a sense of isolation. This is especially the case in winter when mobility might become an issue. A simple thing that atheist communities can do is arrange to provide rides to people, to the grocery store, to doctor's appointments, and to various entertainments. Arranging for transportation or rideshares to events can also go a long way to improving attendance at secular events.

Arranging for regular transportation to major bulk stores like Costco can also be a huge help. Often buying in bulk can be cheaper but can be difficult or impossible for people without transportation. Alternatively, arranging for a delivery service of some kind to pick up and drop off groceries at people's homes would also help a lot.

Hold Food Bank Fundraisers. A lot of people with disabilities will make use of the food bank during their lifetimes. The problem is that food banks are not able to cater to special needs diets. Celiac or gluten allergy? Too bad. Lactose Intolerant? Suck it up. It's not that they don't want to help with those types of diets, but food banks don't receive a lot of options to begin with. If you want as an organization to help people in your community who are struggling, do a money drive and food drive for your local food banks. Help stock them with gluten-free options, get them toiletries, and give them money. Any of these three actions can be a huge help. Many people forget about toiletries when doing food bank drives, but there are many people for whom the only feminine hygiene products they can get are those that come in from time to time.

Start a Meal Program. It can be difficult at times for people struggling with illness to make themselves healthy meals—either due to the effort in standing, lack of energy, or lack of money to buy healthy foods. Regardless of the reason, this is one action that a lot of churches provide that is very useful. Members of the community make extra meals that are then delivered to the needy in the community. At times, the community buys gift cards for local grocery chains to give to people so they can buy food. Either of these options can be a huge help to someone who is struggling.

Start a Visit Program. I've mentioned before the sense of isolation often felt by people struggling with illness and disability. Having a list of people who could use a visit either once a week or once a month from people can go a long way to reducing that sense of isolation. This can be combined with the meal program, or just be organized on its own. This service should be offered to people in the hospital who spend long periods of time by themselves.

Create an Item/Clothes Exchange. One person's trash can be another person's treasure. Having a monthly exchange where people can bring in their old furniture or clothing to be exchanged can be very useful for people who can't afford new things. Having that type of community can also be very helpful when, for example, someone loses their home due to a fire.

Choose Accessible Locations for Events. Having been an organizer myself, I know that securing an ideal location for an event is not always possible. However, I find that often accessibility is the lowest priority for many organizers. Often the excuse is that they never see people in wheelchairs or with canes at their events, ignoring of course that if their events are inaccessible, then of course people with such disabilities wouldn't be there.

Remember, not every person for whom accessibility is an issue is going to be visible. They may not require a cane but have a problem with stairs. They may be able to handle stairs part of the time but not at others.

If your event does have elevator access, make sure they are clearly marked.

Rent a Wheelchair. A couple years ago I helped plan a protest with regard to the unfair jailing of atheist bloggers in Bangladesh. I did so with the expectation that I would be unable to participate since part of the protest included a march of a few kilometers, something that was outside my capabilities. The organization, however, decided to rent a wheelchair for me so that I could be included. It made a huge difference and meant that the protest had one more attendee to add to their numbers. Not everyone who has trouble with mobility will have a wheelchair of their own. They may not even know that renting a wheelchair is an option. By including information about rentals or mentioning that such is available, you open up the possibility of attendance to a lot more people.

Create Disability Scholarships. Many people who struggle with disabilities also struggle with money. This makes it difficult to attend events, conferences, and other networking-type activities. By providing scholarships or reduced cost tickets for people with disabilities, you lower some of the barriers toward attendance.

Make Presentations More Accessible. This is a big one that is often forgotten about. When booking someone for a talk, remind them to make their presentations more accessible. If they are including graphics or pictures, remind them that they have to describe them for people who cannot see. If possible, try to arrange to have sign-language interpreters to make it possible for people with auditory disabilities to attend. If you provide these services, make sure to make it clear by including that information on your advertisements.

Make sure you are aware of the procedures regarding service dogs. Run through them if you see one in the audience to make sure that people with the service dogs don't have to spend all their time reminding people that they should not pet a dog that is wearing its vest.

In registration documents, include a section where people can make their accessibility needs clear.

Schedule More Disability-Themed Presentations. Regardless what community you belong to, disability activism intersects. This is especially true for feminism, race activism, and atheism. The intersections of disability, whether physical or mental, are huge. By creating more awareness, you also increase more people struggling with these problems to get involved in the community. Not to be self-serving, but if you are looking for speakers, I am available for this purpose.

Hire More People with Disabilities. Often when thinking about representation, people forget about those of us struggling with disability. By hiring more people who struggle with mobility, visual or hearing impairments, or chronic illness, you are likely to get a better perspective on how to be more inclusive.

This is not a complete list but includes only a few ideas of what organizations like Center for Inquiry, American Atheists, and others can do to improve accessibility and the lives of disabled people in their own communities.

64 So It Goes

When I first set out to write this book, I was expecting that it wouldn't take me more than a month or so to write. Two years later I sit here having learned more than I ever expected—about disability and about myself. Some of what got in the way was my disability. Writing about some of the most painful moments of my life made me relive those moments— sometimes even physically.

In the time it took me to write this book, I was approved for disability support payments, and I had my gallbladder removed due to recurring pancreatitis.

In the time it took me to write this book, I learned more about what it means to not just live with a disability, but also to be a disability activist, even within the atheist community, where I have seen well-known atheists fail spectacularly on understanding the need for such activism.

In the time it took me to write this book, I had the needed time to really think about why I was writing it.

Some of my goals are noble. If nothing else I hope to raise awareness surrounding what life is like for people with disabilities. To raise awareness of arthritis and chronic pain in young adults. To raise awareness of Crohn's disease. I hope to create a resource for other people struggling with the same or similar disorders. I hope to give doctors insight into what it means to live with the conditions that they diagnose and maybe foster better relationships between the medical service industry and patients. I hope to motivate politicians and activists to start making changes to our society that are so needed to improve the lives of so many.

Some of my motivations are less noble. Like many writers I have a compulsion to tell a story and mine is one that I've been needing to tell for a long time. I need other people to understand what my life is like. I need people to start paying attention.

I need you. You're my only hope.

Acknowledgments

I received the news that my book was going to be published while I was in the hospital being treated for a Crohn's flare. The symbolism and appropriateness of that was not lost on me, and while there wasn't much that could be done to officially celebrate as long as I was on clear liquids only and IVs full of steroids and pain killers, the nurses did their best to congratulate me and make me feel special.

This book was first inspired by an offhand remark by my mother. During the spring and summer when I was desperately seeking answers regarding my leg, my mother was concerned about how reclusive I was becoming. Even though I may not have been open about it, I think it was obvious that I was floundering. It was rapidly becoming clear to me that my life would not follow the pattern that I had expected, even planned for.

I don't remember what brought the subject up, though I do know we were sitting by the kitchen. It wasn't a big thing, just a passing comment that since I liked writing I should write a book about my experiences. That maybe it could help others going through the same thing.

That thought percolated in my mind for several years, and as people began responding positively to my blog, the thoughts became more insistent. Then one day, I couldn't work anymore. My conditions, combined with the stresses surrounding me, got to be too much. I started working on applying for disability.

The process to get on disability takes a long time, and while I waited, the idea of the book came roaring back into my mind. I set up an IndieGoGo campaign to gauge interest. The response was overwhelming. While I didn't make the entire goal, I did receive enough to live on for a few months.

More overwhelming than the monetary support was the influx of messages I received from people who wanted this book to exist.

While originally I hoped that the book would take me only a few weeks to write, it ended up taking me much longer than I expected. A part of the reason for that was that I hadn't expected how much writing about my experiences would force me to relive some of them. Writing about pain, made me feel it. Writing about symptoms, made me more aware of the ones I was having.

I learned a lot about myself and my disability while writing this book. I learned how to listen to my body more, to trust my instincts. Through the lens of hindsight, I was able to see how serious some of what I went through really was. I marveled at how close I had actually come to facing mortality, despite my young age.

I can't say if this book would ever have been written without that offhand remark, and for that I will always be grateful to my mother. No matter what, Mom, you always inspire me to be the best person I can be.

I couldn't have written this book without my amazing wife and partner, Alyssa, who was there for me throughout the whole process. She spent countless hours supplying me with my current caffeine injection method of choice and keeping my spirits up. She was there to comfort me when writing certain scenes made me relive some of the most difficult times in my life. She was there when I was wracked by pain, by tears, by overwhelming sickness, and by doubt. She offered bribes when bribes were needed, tough love when that was needed, and a reminder that what I have to say has value—something I often forget.

She never complained when my current writing sprint kept us eating the same leftovers for a week straight, or even about how much time I spent writing this book at Starbucks.

Without her support, her love, I could not have done this. Alyssa, you are without a doubt my love, my heart, and my strength. Your amazing smile has brought warmth to so many of my days. I love you.

I also want to thank my friends and fellow activists who have acted as my teachers, my sounding board, and my inspiration. You have helped me grow as a person, as an activist, and as a writer. Many of you helped me by answering my seemingly random Facebook questions and offering opinions of various chapters and excerpts. Some of you helped by sharing your own experiences to give me a broader understanding of disability.

Some of you helped by telling me when I was wrong about something, and forced me to rethink things.

Special thanks in particular to Neurodivergent K of Radical Neurodivergence Speaking, an autistic activist who not only helped create a lot of the language being used in different areas of disability activism but who also has been one of the single greatest influences in helping shape my thinking with regard to both disability in general and my own disabilities in particular. She is an inspiration to me and many others, and I hope someday soon the world will recognize the amazing gifts she brings to bear in this fight. And maybe, just maybe, let her have one day or conference that doesn't decide that not trying to kill her is too much of an inconvenience.

I want to thank my wonderful first editors, Marlowe Fillipov and Seanna Watson. Your notes were extremely helpful and helped make a mess of stories into a coherent whole. I also want to thank Greta Christina for providing me with an introduction to my wonderful publisher.

I would also like to thank the people who donated to my fundraiser and made it possible for me to take the time I needed to write this book.

I want to send a special thank you to Elliander Joy Davis, who donated $500 to my campaign, and to Andrew D. Jewell, Michelle Kothe, Simon-Pierre Fortin, Natasha Yar, Seanna and Steve Watson, Sharon Stone, and others who have chosen to remain anonymous, who donated $100 or more to my campaign. Your support went a long way toward making this book a reality, and I sincerely hope that you like the result.

I would like to give a warm wish of thanks to the wonderful Starbucks crews at Trainyards and at Lola. These two shops in particular were my home for many of the weeks I spent writing this book. Not only did they keep the atmosphere pleasant, but they also spent time talking to me when I needed to work out a thought, and I will always appreciate the occasional free drink or upgrade as they helped keep me well supplied in caffeine and distraction.

Finally, I would like to thank everyone who has played a role in my healthcare, especially my wonderful GI, Dr. Sy, who does his best to help me when my body seems determined to make no sense; the wonderful Dr. Karsh, who without a doubt saved my life when he got me the first appointment with Dr. Sy; Dr. Jaroszynska, who started me on the process toward getting real answers about my legs, and without whose referrals and help I would not have regained as much mobility as I have; and all the nurses who have kept me going through difficult admissions and long waits in the ER and observation rooms, and who have helped me advocate to get the care that I need. In a world that more accurately reflected how important certain jobs are, nurses would be paid outrageously well. Their work more than any other is in helping patients. It is their gentle hands that soothe us, their skill and knowledge that protect us, and their compassion that makes dealing with doctors at all possible. I don't have to believe in the supernatural to have met angels; I have done so every time I have been admitted to hospital.

Thank you to my parents who helped pay for my treatment as well as my education. For their help in putting me in contact with doctors who helped, and for trying to learn what it means to have a disabled child. You gave me the skills and strength I needed to do this, through your own example. I hope that one day you will be as proud of me as I am of both of you.

About the Author

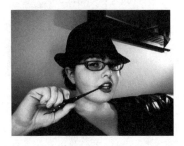

Ania Bula is a disabled, queer, wibbly-wobbly gendery-wendery, social justice activist who is pro-choice, pro–sex work, and manages to say all that in one breath. She writes about a variety of issues including atheism, sex and sexology, psychology, social justice, and her own struggles with body and health issues. She lives in Ottawa with her wife, two cats, three turtles, several fish, and two dogs.